Keeping Up the Good Work:

A Practitioner's Guide to Mental Health Ethics

Second Edition

Leonard J. Haas, PhD
John L. Malouf, PhD

Professional Resource Press
Sarasota, Florida

Published by Professional Resource Press
(An imprint of Professional Resource Exchange, Inc.)
Post Office Box 15560
Sarasota, FL 34277-1560

The copy editor for this book was Patricia Hammond, the managing editor was Debbie Fink, the production coordinator was Laurie Girsch, and the cover designer was Carol Tornatore.

Library of Congress Cataloging-in-Publication Data

Haas, Leonard, J.
    Keeping up the good work : a practitioner's guide to mental health ethics / Leonard J. Haas, John L. Malouf. -- 2nd ed.
        p.   cm.
    Includes bibliographical references and index.
    ISBN 1-56887-012-4
    1. Mental health personnel--Professional ethics. 2. Psychiatric ethics. I. Malouf, John L. II. Title.
    [DNLM: 1. Ethics, Professional. 2. Mental Health Services-
-standards. 3. Professional-Patient Relations. WM 62 H112k 1995]
RC455.2.E8H33   1995
174'.2--dc20
DNLM/DLC
for Library of Congress   94-47583
                                        CIP

Table of Contents

Preface to the First Edition

Although mental health practice has never been simple or stress free, it seems to many of us that the strains are increasing and that the role of mental health practitioners is becoming more complicated, for a number of reasons. First, practitioners are continually faced with the pressures of economic survival, such as receiving third-party reimbursement, collecting from clients, and so on. Compounding this is the recent trend toward managed care health maintenance organizations, preferred provider arrangements, and other alternatives to more traditional forms of reimbursement. Second, the aftermath of such legal decisions as *Tarasoff* has placed practitioners in a quandary regarding who their clients are and to whom they may be obligated. For example, if we report a potentially dangerous client, we run the risk of being held liable for breaking confidentiality. If we fail to report, we run the risk of being held liable for not protecting the public. Significant increases in malpractice insurance premiums provide evidence of a more litigious society, and suggest that the level of paranoia among professionals may be at least partly justified. Such challenges have complicated the already difficult task of understanding and modifying human behavior.

When confronted by this multiplicity of demands and obligations, practitioners unfortunately may neglect to pay adequate attention to the ethical standards and values that should guide their practice. Instead, we may compromise or confuse such standards in the face of more immediate practical, financial, or legal considerations. The practice of giving a client a diagnosis because it is reimbursable by insurance companies; accepting an individual as a client, even though one has no demonstrable competence in treating the problem presented; and "ethics" workshops that are in reality aimed at avoiding lawsuits are all examples of situations in which ethical considerations are sacrificed for the sake of other requirements. Even in the best of circumstances, the ethical course of action is often not easy or clear-cut.

Our motivation for writing this book was to help clinical practitioners understand and apply ethical principles in their practices. The various topics we cover represent those areas of professional practice where ethical concerns are dominant or where practitioners commonly misunderstand their ethical obligations or options.

We are aware that much of what has been written concerning professional ethics has been so general and theoretical that it is difficult for the practitioner to apply. In response to this limitation, we have attempted to apply solid ethical principles to the practical problems professionals face daily. While many, if not most, ethical problems defy hard and fast rules, several chapters in this book present relevant questions or guidelines that practitioners should consider in making a decision. The guidelines aim to focus the reader's attention on relevant issues and aid in decision making. Some of what we have written may seem to simply represent common knowledge or good judgment. Nonetheless, much "common knowledge" is overlooked in the course of a busy practice. We hope that by reading and thinking about these issues, practitioners will be more deliberate in their practical decisions. We have also tried to maintain a helpful and positive attitude. Such an orientation reflects our belief that the vast majority of mental health professionals sincerely want to provide ethical services, as well as make a reasonable living and avoid lawsuits.

This is not a book on legalities, although legal considerations will be considered where appropriate in the light of the ethical issue being discussed. This is not a book on professionalism, although there are numerous occasions when making ethical decisions will bear upon aspects of professionalism. Nor is this a book on clinical strategies, although making ethical decisions clearly has a substantial effect on practitioners' clinical strategies. Our hope, rather, is that in making clinical decisions of various sorts, readers will consider not only what is legally, practically, and clinically justified, but also what is ethical. Thus, we hope that through reading this book, practitioners will integrate higher levels of ethical behavior into their practices.

Further, this is not a book written solely for psychologists, despite the fact that both of the authors are psychologists. Rather, we address this work to all clinical practitioners in the mental health professions. Although there are certain distinct differences in training, expertise, and prerogatives among the various professions, in practice there are many more similarities than differences. All of the mental health disciplines share a sense of professionalism, a duty to provide for the welfare of clients or patients, and a commitment to improving standards of practice, among other things. We hope that this book will be useful both in graduate coursework and in professional development, to social workers, psychiatrists, marriage and family therapists, and other mental health workers in addition to psychologists.

It would be unethical for us to fail to acknowledge with gratitude the contributions of many people to the successful completion of this book. First, we wish to thank Rob Showell and Brenda Goates, our indefatigable typists, who labored with us through many revisions of this manuscript. We also wish to acknowledge the help and considerate prodding of our publishers Peter Keller and Larry Ritt. Thanks are due as well to Samuel Knapp for his constructive and helpful review of the manuscript. We dedicate this book to our families - Rudy and Gerda Haas, Abby Gottsegen, Bea and Phelon Malouf, Molly Malouf, and Emily Malouf for their support and love during this process.

Preface to the Second Edition

In the 5 years that have gone by since the first edition of this book, the world of the mental health professional has become more complex, from an ethical as well as from a clinical standpoint. Prior to the publication of the first edition, the watershed for the field of mental health was the *Tarasoff* decision; the trend to enlarge clinicians' responsibilities for the potential actions of their clients has continued and in some ways accelerated since *Tarasoff*. Now there is yet another major upheaval that expands therapists' responsibilities: the advent of managed care reimbursement schemes. It remains to be seen whether the "managed care revolution" will have the same impact on the ethics and standards of the mental health professions as did the *Tarasoff* decision and its progeny. Nonetheless it is undeniable that the rise of utilization reviewers, quality assurance schemes, preauthorization requirements, and increasing demands for disclosure of records will have an enormous impact on the way psychotherapists practice.

A second and more encouraging trend that was apparent to us in 1989 has continued to accelerate; that is the seriousness with which the mental health professions take their ethical responsibilities. All the codes of the major mental health professions have been revised, some quite substantially, since the publication of the first edition. The codes have become less abstract and more detailed. Although some would argue that these have shifted our codes of professional conduct from ethics codes to legal practice guidelines, the fact remains that statements of professional principles by and large are articulated more clearly and possible ramifications better explored.

What else has been happening since 1989? Among the major trends in professional ethics has been the recognition that multiple relationships remain hazardous, and that exceptional care must be taken to avoid becoming ethically mired in them. The rise of HIV and AIDS has raised ethical questions about the extension of the duty to protect and the degree to which confidentiality should be protected. As noted previously, the rise of managed care plans and health care reform has made more complicated the carrying out of the clinician's fiduciary responsibilities to his or her clients.

This second edition deals with all of these emerging areas of professional ethics. In addition, we include consideration of certain topics which were not covered in the first edition. These include access to clinical information by family members of the mentally ill, the role of the mental health professional in the courtroom, and issues related to abandonment. Whereas some chapters have stood the test of time since the first edition, many chapters have been substantially revised. We have included the most recent revisions of the ethical codes of all the major mental health professions, and we have discussed their implications for practice. As with the first edition, our attempt has been to raise issues of ethics and professional standards in a practical context and with respect for the realities of clinical practice.

The world of the psychotherapist has certainly become more complex in the half decade since the publication of the first edition. A troubling aspect of the rise of new health care reimbursement schemes and the increased competition among mental health professionals is that it is easier than ever to lose sight of professional ethics in the fight for economic survival. Yet we still believe, as we did in 1989, that an effective and economically viable practice can be well guided by the ethics of the mental health professions, and that with the development of "professional character," the psychotherapist can incorporate his or her profession's standards in a way that makes it easier to survive the pressures of legalisms, financial lures, and so on. We hope that this book contributes some small degree of clarity to the continuing dialogue about ethical responsibilities and responsible practice.

We offer it recognizing that the ethical practice of mental health work is not easy, and yet at the same time is exceptionally rewarding.

This revised edition is dedicated to two important people who have joined our nuclear families since the book was originally published: Margot Haas, born March 2, 1993, and Carol Malouf, born much earlier.

Keeping Up the Good Work:

A Practitioner's Guide to Mental Health Ethics

Second Edition

Chapter 1

The Nature of
Professional Ethics

This chapter provides a brief discussion of the theory and philosophy underlying the practice of professional ethics. It deals with three questions: What is professional ethics? What makes an action ethical? Are there different types of ethical obligations?

WHAT IS ETHICS?

One useful method for distinguishing ethics from other major standards for determining whether an action is right, good, or proper is to contrast it with those frameworks. Law (especially criminal law) and etiquette can be thought of as domains similar to ethics, because each focuses on aspects of proper or correct behavior and each specifies penalties for deviation.

Although each set of standards reflects in some respects the consensus of the society or culture that promotes it, moral frameworks are (or should be) developed largely through rational processes. Legal standards, on the other hand, are predominantly developed through political processes, and norms of etiquette are developed for the most part by historical precedent.

Ethical standards, in theory at least, focus on behavior and on motivations that aim at the highest ideals of human behavior. Criminal law, in contrast, focuses primarily on proscribed behavior that may harm other members of the society, and etiquette focuses on behavior that establishes one's good standing within a sub-group.

Actions that violate moral or ethical standards can result in censure, guilt, or social criticism. Illegal behavior, on the other hand, results in actual punishment, if detected; impolite behavior results in social penalties: ostracism or perhaps mild social criticism.

In the view of many moral philosophers, ethics is distinguished by three main features: (a) it is based on *principles*, (b) the principles have *universality* (e.g., could be applied generally to all similar persons), and (c) appropriate behavior may be deduced from the principles by *reasoning*. Thus, ethics proper should involve adherence to a consistent set of principles assumed to be relevant for all individuals in similar situations, which result (deductively) in obligations to take particular actions.

Two relevant facts follow from this. First, codes of professional ethics are actually not pure ethics, but rather a combination of ethics, law, and etiquette; and second, no existing ethical theory (especially no theory of professional ethics) meets the standard set forth above. Thus we are dealing with a somewhat indeterminate, evolving framework with which to guide decisions and actions. Despite this uncertainty, however, a code of professional ethics can indeed provide important guidance in developing one's model of good professional functioning.

THE NATURE OF PROFESSIONAL ETHICS

Although some may argue that professional ethics are distinct from general moral obligations (Beauchamp & Childress, 1979), it is clear that professionals (whether psychologists, psychiatrists, architects, lawyers, or marriage and family therapists) take on special duties to persons who enter professional relationships with them. Legally, the special obligations of the professional are known as *fiduciary*. This term denotes the special duty to care for the welfare of those who have become one's clients or patients. The fact that the mental health practitioner is in a fiduciary relationship with clients implies to some writers that there are special ethical obligations. One example concerns loyalty; the psychotherapist cannot simply decide that he or she is no longer interested in treating a particular patient and discontinue treatment, because this could constitute *abandonment*. This standard of loyalty is higher than that to which average citizens are held, because average citizens are free to terminate most voluntary relationships, such as friendships.

THE NATURE OF ETHICAL ACTS

As noted, actions are generally considered to be ethical if they have the following characteristics: First, they are *principled*; that is, the actor must be able to justify his or her actions in the light of some specific, generally accepted moral principles (e.g., honesty, duty to avoid harming others, respect for human dignity, preservation of freedom). Second, the action must be a *reasoned* outcome of consideration of the principles. This relates to the notion of free will in moral responsibility; that is, the actor is assumed to be capable of choice and thus responsible for basing his or her actions on ethical principles. Third, the action must be *universalizable*; that is, the actor must be able to recommend that others in similar situations do the same thing.

MAJOR TYPES OF ETHICAL JUSTIFICATIONS

TELEOLOGICAL JUSTIFICATION

Although the foregoing suggests that the inherent *features* of certain acts mark them as ethical, the question of their *consequences* can also be raised in this regard. The method of moral justification called *teleology* or *utilitarianism* indicates that an action is ethical if it results in the creation of more good than harm, or as Bentham (1863/1948) phrased it in his famous maxim, produces "the greatest good for the greatest number." This principle has been criticized by ethical theorists because it may lead to "the ends justifying the means." Such criticisms of teleology frequently are based on *deontological* principles. Additional problems with teleological analyses focus on the problem of who is entitled to judge the "good" or "bad" that flows from a moral choice.

DEONTOLOGICAL JUSTIFICATION

Deontology, a contrasting framework with which to justify the ethical quality of actions, posits that actions are ethical if they manifest one of a small set of primary moral characteristics. For example, in early versions of medical ethics, the preservation of life was the primary ethical principle. Thus, an action that was intended to preserve life was ethical regardless of what other consequences it produced. Using a deontological method of determining the rightness of one's actions becomes difficult when more than one moral principle is involved, because deontology provides no decision rules for selecting the more ethical action when each choice is based on a different moral ground. For example, if telling the truth would result in someone's death (the famous example is that of the hospital administrator in Nazi-occupied Europe who is asked if there are any Jewish patients in the hospital), which is the proper course - to be honest or to preserve life? Criticisms of deontological methods of ethical justification focus on this problem, of deontologically ethical actions creating evil results, as a demonstration of the inadequacy of the method.

VARIETIES OF ETHICAL OBLIGATIONS

Ethical obligations can be more or less explicit, and can constitute either the minimally acceptable standard or the ideal to which the ethically responsible practitioner aspires. Minimal standards (the "floor" of ethics) are known as mandatory ethical obligations. Ideals (or the "ceiling" of ethics) are known as aspirational obligations (Gerts, 1981). Generally, one can be criticized or punished for violating mandatory obligations; additionally, one is typically not praised for successfully upholding them. Conversely, individuals are not commonly censured or punished for violating aspirational obligations; much more commonly, those who succeed in upholding such standards are commended and admired. In terms familiar to readers of the Ten Commandments, mandatory obligations can be thought of as "thou shalt nots," whereas aspirational obligations can be thought of as "thou shalts." For example, the *Ethical Principles of Psychologists and Code of Conduct* (American Psychological Association, 1992) has as one of its mandatory ethical obligations the duty to refrain from "uninvited in-person solicitation of business" from potential clients. This injunction is based on the notion that the vulnerabilities of laypersons could be exploited by a mental health professional subtly or directly indicating the presence of a psychological problem. This can be seen as a "thou shalt not." It would be remarkable for a psychologist to be praised for avoiding such solicitation; on the other hand, it would be quite likely that such a practitioner would be censured for participating in such activities. Conversely, the principle embodied in the *Ethical Principles of Psychologists and Code of Conduct* to "promote human dignity" can be seen as an aspirational ethical obligation. It is difficult to determine when a professional has met this obligation, and it could easily be argued that the aim is never completely realized. Indeed, the conscientious practitioner devotes his or her entire professional career to achieving this end. Thus, it would be unusual for a practitioner to be censured for "failing to promote human dignity," whereas it would be much more common for a practitioner who exemplified exceptional ability to promote human dignity to be honored for this.

It is important not to confuse aspirational and mandatory obligations. If one believes that aspirational obligations are in fact mandatory (i.e., mistakes the ethical "ceiling" for the ethical "floor"), one runs the risk of feeling hopelessly inadequate as an ethical practitioner. This approach is not uncommonly seen among professionals in training when they are first exposed to education in professional ethics. They begin to believe that their obligations are so massive and overwhelming as to prevent them from ever functioning effectively as clinicians. Indeed, an important aspect of one's development as a competent, ethical mental health practitioner demands that one be continually aware of aspirational obligations, while at the same time avoiding the overwhelming sense of inadequacy that prevents experiencing any satisfaction with one's work.

Conversely, one can run the risk of confusing mandatory with aspirational obligations (i.e., mistaking the ethical "floor" for the ethical "ceiling"). In such cases the practitioner believes that even the explicitly stated prohibitions in his or her ethical code are simply ideals to be aspired to; failure to uphold these standards is seen as justified if one has made a "good effort." This approach can be seen as a form of rationalization for failure to exert the considerable self-discipline required to act in a professionally responsible manner.

It is also useful to note that ethical obligations leave a tremendous amount of latitude to the judgment of the practitioner. Perhaps this is as it should be, because, as noted before, ethical behavior is based in large part on the practitioner's *choices*. Further, the domains in which mental health practitioners claim expertise are ones that deeply affect the lives of those who call upon us for help. There are many ways to effectively help, and a range of choices that respect individuals' personhood. It is to finding such effective modes of practicing that the remainder of this book is devoted.

Chapter 2

A Framework for
Ethical Decision Making

As we have suggested, no ethical practitioner (indeed, no professional practitioner at all) can avoid making choices; the provision of ethically appropriate and clinically sound services requires constant and careful decision making. These deliberations about the ethically appropriate course of action may be excruciating in their detail or quite fleeting, incorporated almost automatically into ongoing professional activities. The central ethical aspects of a particular problem may be immediately evident or highly subtle, and the relevant professional standards may be clear-cut in their implications for action or frustratingly vague in providing guidance.

The purpose of this chapter is to present an explicit framework for ethical decision making. This framework is not intended to be rigorously followed each time an ethical question arises. Rather, it is an attempt to make explicit what should "naturally" occur in the course of deciding on an ethically appropriate action in practice. As we learn more about expertise in general, we find that highly skilled practitioners integrate an enormous amount of information in the context of underlying "operating principles" regularly in the course of their work (Patel & Groen, 1991). Generally, the practitioner's intuitive sense of the right decision (assuming proper training in competent professional service) will facilitate the decision-making process. However, as the ethical dimensions of practice become increasingly important and complex, attending to less obvious aspects of the decision-making process becomes vital.

In what follows, we briefly summarize the major "information gathering" aspects of the process of making ethical decisions; we then present a sequential decision-making process and describe its possible uses.

PHASES OF INFORMATION GATHERING

This section describes three domains in which the practitioner must gather information before actually making a decision. Each area of information gathering can be conducted in more or less detail. One's information gathering may be as simple as mentally reviewing the relevant aspects of the situation, or it may be as complex as reviewing the literature, consulting with colleagues, and requesting professional opinions from philosophers, lawyers, or others. Briefly, the clinician must identify three elements before being able to make an ethical decision: (a) the nature of the ethical problem; (b) the identities and preferences of those persons who have a legitimate stake in the outcome of the problem (the "stake-holders"); and (c) the relevant professional and legal standards (if any) that bear on the case at hand. More detailed discussion of each of these domains follows.

IDENTIFYING THE ETHICAL PROBLEM

The first question in the initial analysis of a particular case is, what makes this an ethical dilemma? Not all problems are ethical; some are simply technical. For example, a practitioner may wish to determine the best method for treating migraine headaches. This is a technical decision and not (unless unusual circumstances exist) an ethical one. Conversely, deciding whether or not to inform the fiancée of a patient that her intended has episodic rage reactions *does* involve an ethical decision.

The key questions for the practitioner are, first, is there an ethical problem or problems? Second, if more than one ethical problem exists, which is the most important? It is important to note with regard to this second issue that the tendency to proliferate dilemmas is always present. If at all possible, it is helpful to reduce the ethical dimensions of a situation to one or two primary ethical questions. Third, if an ethical dilemma can be identified, is there a way to resolve it without choosing between competing ethical principles? This is an important avenue in the initial decision-making process, in that some ethical dilemmas can be reduced to technical problems simply by finding a method of operating that eliminates the conflict. For example, there is a potential conflict between the preservation of confidentiality when treating a minor client (for example, an adolescent) and the legitimate demands of a worried parent to know what is happening in therapy. This can be a painful ethical dilemma, but therapists who work with children can routinely obtain permission from the parents of minors in advance (or at least discuss the issue openly before a crisis arises) so that the ethical dilemma does not arise.

IDENTIFYING LEGITIMATE STAKE-HOLDERS

In the ideal case (which almost never exists), the only parties legitimately concerned with the outcome of an ethical dilemma would be the practitioner and the client. In practice, however, other parties are typically involved. Increasingly, the party paying for mental health services is not the party receiving them. Such situations include cases in which the clinician is employed by an institution to render services, cases in which services are paid for by a third party, and cases in which a third party (such as an employer, parent, or court officer) legitimately orders professional services to be provided. It is important for the clinician to be clear about who has a legitimate right to be taken into account in making clinical decisions. The notion that some parties have legitimate stakes in the outcomes of a situation implies that their preferences about those outcomes should be taken into account. Once the identity of the stake-holders has been determined, some attempt to ascertain their preferences must be made.

In certain situations the problem is of such magnitude that parties not directly involved in contracting for the service have a legitimate stake in the outcome as well. In particular, it is at times essential to consider the interests of future members of the same class of consumer, unidentifiable members of society who may be affected by the outcome of the case, the practitioner's profession as a whole (and its image in the eyes of the public), and - most broadly - the general social climate in a particular society.

Thus, for example, decisions to breach or not to breach confidentiality may in part rest on considerations of the public's general level of trust in the mental health professions. Likewise, the decision to deceive or not to deceive a particular consumer about diagnosis or treatment plan may contribute to the general public distrust of professionals, or a generally lowered level of respect for individuals in society.

The foregoing should also imply that the clinicians themselves are among the legitimate stake-holders in the delivery of mental health services. Stated more plainly, this implies that the practitioner's preferences may also be taken into account.

Even though ethical decision making is sometimes presented as a purely cognitive or rational activity, it is important to recognize that there is a strong emotional or aesthetic component to most ethical decisions. Ideally, such subjective preferences flow from a professional history of making ethical choices and carefully considering the contribution one's actions make to human welfare. Unfortunately, there can also arise situations in which a practitioner deduces from the applicable principles that a particular course of action is mandated but feels that it would not be "right" to engage in it. In such cases, reflection and consultation are called for. In the best outcome, either one's personal ethical standards or one's degree of comfort with sound ethical choices would evolve and mature.

IDENTIFYING RELEVANT STANDARDS

Although we have until this point described the ethical dimension of professional decision making as almost entirely involving moral principles, the society at large has taken intense interest in professional self-regulation. As a result, choices that in the past might have been made entirely on moral grounds ("Is this good?") are increasingly being made on mandatory grounds ("Is there a rule mandating or prohibiting this?"). Mental health practice, applied philosophy, and legal theory have become increasingly focused on the standards of practice as clients have shown their willingness to use legal power to enforce their views of appropriate professional actions. This in turn has led to the evolution of professional ethical codes into standards of practice. Precedents have emerged that mandate particular actions in particular situations. These precedents or standards may not always be clear-cut; however, once they exist in at least partially codified form, the responsible practitioner must have a good reason for *not* adhering to them. Frequently, the existing standards are vague in their specifications for action. This does allow the practitioner to decide what the range of choices consistent with a given standard might be. For example, at the broadest level the social workers' *Code of Ethics* (National Association of Social Workers, 1993) mandates that social workers act to promote human welfare. The literal interpretation of this varies with the situation and with the specifics of the case.

An additional rule of thumb that may help in the identification of relevant standards is that one should not fear consultation in these matters. It is often unclear which, if any, existing professional standard bears on a specific case; consulting with experienced colleagues or experts in the particular area may help clarify the situation.

THE PROCESS OF
ETHICAL DECISION MAKING

Once practitioners have gathered enough information to believe that they can adequately identify the ethical nature of the problems that face them, the legitimately involved parties, and the existing standards, they are in a position to begin arriving at a decision. This section describes a sequential process of establishing that an ethical decision has been made. It draws on a number of sources including material by Rest (1982), Jonsen, Siegler, and Winslade (1982), and Candee (1985). In the most general terms, this ethical decision-making framework rests on three underlying presumptions: the dignity and free will of the individual (autonomy), the obligation of professionals to respect the existing standards and expectations of the society that legitimizes their activities (responsibility), and the duty to avoid special or self-serving interpretations or situations (universality). In its simplest form the framework is presented as a flow chart in Figure 1 (p. 13). Discussions of various phases of the flow chart follow.

DOES A RELEVANT PROFESSIONAL, LEGAL, OR SOCIAL STANDARD EXIST?

As implied in the preceding section, this question obligates the psychologist to engage in the common professional activity of literature review, consultation with respected colleagues, or both. The nature of standards that may be accessed to answer this question range from the highly specific (e.g., *Standards for Educational and Psychological Testing* [American Educational Research Association et al., 1985] which mandates specific aspects of testing procedure) to the quite broad (e.g., the general social standard that one should keep one's promises, sometimes also codified in legal statutes that make fraud a criminal offense).

IS THERE A REASON TO DEVIATE FROM THE STANDARD?

Two types of cases may reduce the usefulness of existing standards. First, the existing standard may be so vague as to prevent its being used in a particular case. Second, the specifics of a given case may lead to more harm than benefit being produced by adhering to the standard (this is actually a special case of conflicting standards, because the overriding ethical obligation of all the mental health professions is to promote human welfare). An example of this question in use involves a case in which the mother of a 32-year-old patient being seen by a psychotherapist calls for information about her child.* A standard for this kind of case exists; the practitioner is obligated to uphold confidentiality. However, assume that in this case there is risk of suicide on the part of the patient. Then there may be a good reason to deviate from the professional standard in the interests of protecting patient

---

*Names and all identifying characteristics of persons in all case examples have been disguised thoroughly to protect privacy.

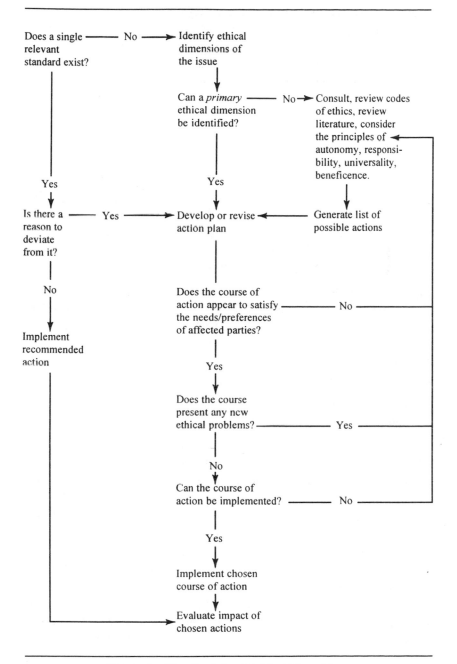

Figure 1.　The Decision-Making Flow Chart.

welfare (however, note that this ethical dilemma may be resolved, if there is sufficient time, by contacting the patient and obtaining permission, even if it is not strictly required, before revealing information to the parent).

WHAT ARE THE ETHICAL DIMENSIONS OF THE ISSUE?

If there is no single ethical standard or principle that pertains, the practitioner must identify the significant ethical issues. That is, what are the dimensions that make the issue problematic? For instance, is there a conflict between a need to preserve confidentiality and a need to protect the public? Mandatory child abuse reporting statutes frequently are used to illustrate this problem. On the one hand, it is argued that reporting suspected child abuse will drive out of treatment individuals who need it in order to parent their children effectively. On the other hand, it is argued that to fail to report exposes the child in the family to the risk that the psychotherapist will not be able to affect the parent's acting out. The standard method of resolving this conflict involves the invocation of informed consent: The prospective client is informed at the outset of treatment that information regarding the possible abuse of a child must be reported. However, this solution raises another problem: Will the potentially abusive parent be encouraged to suppress information and thereby not get treatment for a significant problem? This presents a conflict between the obligation to honestly inform the prospective client about treatment and the obligation to provide competent service for the important problems. As another example, a clinical intervention that has been shown effective for a particular problem may be one that is rendered less effective the more the client knows about it (e.g., paradoxical intervention). Often, when the appropriate course of action is unclear, it is because of competing ethical principles; they must be defined and classified in order for there to be a chance to reconcile them.

CAN A PRIMARY ETHICAL DIMENSION BE SPECIFIED?

In cases such as the preceding, an overriding principle can often be identified. For example, legal and ethical principles indicate that when clear and present danger exists, the obligation to protect potential victims overrides the obligation to uphold clients' understanding that the practitioner will keep information private. From a teleological perspective, this concept rests on the predictability of harm: The chances that harm will come to an individual who is being threatened by a potentially violent patient are greater than the chances that the patient will be harmed by the disclosure. Indeed, some commentators have suggested that truly benefiting a potentially violent patient involves helping them to avoid acting on their violent impulses.

GENERATE A LIST OF POSSIBLE ACTIONS

In cases when no single ethical dimension outweighs all others, a variety of actions may prove to be ethically appropriate. As in other problem-solving situations, a "solution-generating" or "brainstorming" phase can be helpful. In this phase, the practitioner may benefit from reading relevant ethical codes, reviewing legal statutes, or consulting with colleagues. It is not always necessary to determine which ethical principle is dominant. Rather, time should be spent devising solutions that reconcile competing principles. Novel, creative solutions and ways to reconcile competing principles should be explored. For instance, in the case of the conflict between informed consent versus competence mentioned in connection with paradoxical therapy, the practitioner may be able to find a way to protect the client's right to know about treatment procedures without compromising the effectiveness of the intervention. Some authors have argued that this may be accomplished by providing some general information about treatment (appropriate to the client's level of sophistication) and allowing the client to ask for further information as needed. Others have argued that paradox works regardless of the level of awareness possessed by the client (Hunsley, 1988).

Following the brainstorming phase, a cost-benefit analysis should be conducted. Each alternative should be evaluated in terms of its potential benefits and potential costs. The needs of the client as well as the needs of other associated individuals (such as family members), the public, and the mental health profession should be considered. The alternative that results in an optimum resolution for the greatest number of interested parties should be chosen.

DOES THE NEW COURSE OF ACTION APPEAR TO SATISFY THE NEEDS/PREFERENCES OF AFFECTED PARTIES?

Although the ethical codes of most mental health disciplines underline the general obligation to promote human welfare, in particular cases this always translates into promoting the interests of one or more involved parties. Thus, if no standard exists with regard to a particular dilemma, or there is good reason to deviate from existing standards because they seem inadequate to deal with the facts of the case, a course of action that takes into account (better yet, satisfies) the needs and preferences of affected parties must be developed. The notion here is that, all other things being equal, the practitioner is obliged to render the services that he or she has agreed to provide. Typically, the services are provided to satisfy some need of the consumer.

DOES THE COURSE OF ACTION PRESENT ANY NEW ETHICAL PROBLEMS?

This question is raised because of the nature of ethical decisions. Specifically, a major question that must be asked of any course of action to have it qualify as ethical is that of universalizability, as noted previously. In other words: Would I recommend this same course of action to every other person essentially similar to me who is operating in essentially the same circumstances? This is a more limited version of the question: Would you recommend that everybody do this? This notion of universalizability is what distinguishes ethical action from expedient action. An example of this question involves a case in which the patient of a psychotherapist is involved in a relationship the therapist considers extremely unhealthy. The therapist is in a position to be able to tell a "credible lie" to the patient regarding the behavior of her partner. The therapist believes that this action would be for the best interest of the patient. Is this an ethical course of action? We would argue that it is not, because the therapist could not reasonably expect that everyone in a similar situation should engage in a lie (thereby possibly reducing or damaging the trust the patient has in the therapist). Thus, the decision to lie would be seen as one of expediency rather than one of ethical responsibility. Another example involves the question of whether a clinician should accept a gift from a client. Assessing whether or not one would suggest the same course of action to other practitioners in the same situation clarifies the issue dramatically.

It is also a characteristic of ethical actions that they are based on principles. In the ideal case, the actor can specify the principles on which the course of action is based. A colloquial way of describing this element of the process has been proposed by D. Callahan (personal communication, 1980). It is the "clean, well-lit room" standard. That is, could the practitioner's decision be comfortably defended to a group of his or her peers? Although some unethical decisions could pass this standard, no ethical decision should fail it.

CAN THE COURSE OF ACTION BE IMPLEMENTED?

This question has two parts: It refers to issues of practicality and to issues of prudence. Practicality refers simply to the possibility that one could actually put the course of action into effect. Actions that involve social reform, changes in social policy, and massive upheavals in common ways of practice are unlikely to be implementable in a particular case. For example, suggesting to a depressed homemaker that she become more politically active and more conscious of her gender-based oppression would be considered (at least in the case of a patient who appears untroubled by her role choice) more likely to be a long-range political remedy rather than an implementable course of action.

The "prudence" aspect of this question refers simply to the fact that ethical decisions may at times be costly to the practitioner who implements them. This question is simply to draw the practitioner's attention to the fact that effort and cost may be involved in implementing a decision, and these issues should be thought through in advance. This sort of situation arises, for example, when a professional in training believes that a supervisor is acting unethically and wishes to confront him or her. As we comment later, there are alternatives to an immediate confrontation that would be potentially less damaging to one's training or career.

IMPLEMENT THE CHOSEN COURSE OF ACTION

This recommendation appears straightforward but does involve other (nonethical) skills such as assertiveness, tenacity, the existence of a supportive social network, and the ability to communicate one's chosen action in noncondescending and humane terms. For example, psychologists are obligated to terminate a professional relationship when it is no longer beneficial to the consumer (American Psychological Association, 1992). It is sometimes the case that psychotherapists derive tremendous enjoyment from working with particular clients, and some clients, when confronted with the idea of termination, will resist and object to this. Nonetheless, despite the emotional difficulty of implementing such a decision, it truly is the ethical course of action (at least in the case where no benefit seems to be accruing to the client).

CONSULT AND REVIEW CODES OF ETHICS; REVIEW LITERATURE; CONSIDER ETHICAL PRINCIPLES

This implies that the practitioner has available resources (such as information, time, and energy) to review and extract usable information about ethical dilemmas. Other sections of this book will indicate possible resources that may help in this task, but it should be made clear that this task is more easily written about than performed.

LIMITATIONS OF THE FRAMEWORK

A limitation inherent in this framework is that it is quite general. In the chapters to come it should be clear that many specific situations have already been discussed, written about, and occasionally studied empirically. In these domains there may be perhaps fewer questions, but no matter how much ethical theorizing and ethical research goes on, the constantly evolving nature of professional practice will always produce cases with unique features that puzzle practitioners. The framework presented herein is simply to guide the practitioner in developing perspective on such puzzling cases.

There are other limitations of this (and any) decision-making framework. First, since a decision-making framework is based on rationality, there is no way to completely eliminate the possibility of self-serving rationalization. Second, the framework proposed above does not thoroughly take into account legal considerations. More generally, this may be considered as an issue of prudence. Is it prudent for a clinician to reason purely on the basis of ethical considerations without regard for legal liability or existing legal precedent? The answer is no. However, as a first step it is useful to consider the purely ethical or purely moral aspects of decision making. The prudential elements of the process can then be considered (as was briefly noted) under the question of implementability.

Finally, the proposed framework makes no allowances for ambiguity or mistakes; certainly these occur. It is in the nature of ethically responsible practice that one is not held blameworthy if one attempted to act appropriately and do what one thought was best. However, it is also ethically incumbent on the responsible practitioner to learn from his or her mistakes.

Chapter 3

Competence in Clinical Practice

The expectation that clinicians will deliver competent service is fundamental to the notion of professional mental health practice. This is borne out by the codes of ethics of the various mental health disciplines, which contain numerous prominent statements focused on the issue of competence. For instance, the *Ethical Principles of Psychologists and Code of Conduct* (American Psychological Association, 1992) states, "Psychologists . . . recognize the boundaries of their particular competencies and the limitations of their expertise. They provide only those services and use only those techniques for which they are qualified by education, training, or experience" (Principle A). The social workers' *Code of Ethics* (National Association of Social Workers [NASW], 1993) states, "The social worker should strive to become and remain proficient in professional practice and the performance of professional functions" (Principle B). The *Code of Ethics* of the American Association for Marriage and Family Therapy (AAMFT, 1991) asserts "Marriage and family therapists maintain high standards of professional competence and integrity" (Principle 3). *The Principles of Medical Ethics With Annotations Especially Applicable to Psychiatry* (American Psychiatric Association, 1993), states, "A physician shall be dedicated to providing competent medical service with compassion and respect for human dignity" (§1).

Although the preceding statements, along with many others, underscore the importance of delivering competent service to patients or clients, defining what that competence consists of may be quite difficult.

Interestingly, at its root, competence is related to competition. Competence stems from the roots *com*, together, and *peter*, to seek: hence, to strive together or seek (Webster, 1956, p. 370). Consideration of the typical threshold for competent practice seems to rest on this aspect of the definition; that is, more psychologists than we would like to admit seem to consider themselves competent if they can match the abilities of "the competition." This might be considered the lowest common denominator standard for competence. Moving from a consideration of the roots of the term to its actual definition, however, shows that competence means "capacity equal to requirement; adequate fitness or ability" (Webster, 1956, p. 370). In law, competence is defined as "legal . . . qualification, . . . power, or fitness" to do something (Webster, 1956, p. 370). Thus our analysis must focus on what it is that mental health practitioners are called upon to do. Also, professional competence includes both declarative expertise ("knowing what") and procedural expertise ("knowing how") (Faust, 1986).

Some might argue that attainment of competence occurs through obtaining the relevant credentials. However, although credentials are a necessary condition to practice, they are not sufficient to establish professional competence. Credentials per se do not guarantee competence, although presumably the lack of credentials would be a strong indicator of incompetence to perform certain professional activities.

It could also be inferred from the various professions' ethical codes that whenever practitioners violate an ethical principle they can be said to have acted in an incompetent manner. Indeed, it may be asserted that *all* ethical principles can be derived from the principle of competence. Yet to define competence in this way makes the concept equivalent to the tenet of medical ethics: "above all, do no harm." Although this is likely to generate little disagreement, it also leaves unenlightened the practitioner who wants to do some good (consistent with other tenets of all codes of professional ethics). Thus, this chapter discusses a more usable definition of competence, derived in part from concepts advanced by Wiens (1983), Haas (1993), Keith-Spiegel and Koocher (1985), and others.

Competence consists of appropriate professional education and training, continuing education, willingness to subject decisions to peer review, openness to criticism by colleagues, willingness to confess ignorance or error when appropriate, and concentrated and sustained efforts to deepen one's clinical craftsmanship (Pellegrino, 1979). Keith-Spiegel and Koocher (1985) emphasize as an aspect of competence the recognition of *limitations* in one's abilities as well as knowing one's strengths and skills.

Stated differently, a competent clinician is one who has the requisite *knowledge* to understand and conceptualize a particular clinical issue, the necessary *skills* to apply this knowledge in effective ways, and the *judgment* to use such knowledge and skills. Put yet another way, the competent clinician knows what to do, how to do it, and when to do it. For example, a therapist who uses a heavily confrontational style of treatment with a prepsychotic individual may possess extensive knowledge about the technique but may lack judgment about the most appropriate situations in which to use it.

As this discussion implies, a major aspect of *professional* mental health practice is the moral obligation on the individual professional to insure the quality of service. Currently, however, government (primarily at the state level), as the protector of potential patients, has become reluctant to rely solely on practitioners' ethics to guarantee competent treatment. Instead, for the purpose of protecting the public, legal standards of minimum competence have been established (and are constantly in the process of being refined). Although this chapter deals in part with legal standards of minimum competence, our purpose is primarily to help the practitioner put the issue of competence into perspective in his or her own practice.

LICENSURE

The primary legal vehicle by which the public is protected from incompetent practice is licensure. All states have provisions for the licensure or certification of at least some mental health professions, but the question of the role of licensure in guaranteeing competent therapeutic service is nonetheless still hotly debated. The process has been criticized (e.g., Bernstein & LeComte, 1981; Gross, 1978) and defended (e.g., Kane, 1982; Wiens, 1983) extensively in the literature.   An extended discussion of licensure is beyond the scope of this book (cf. Fretz & Mills, 1980, for a review); however, there exist some issues regarding licensure that are relevant for the present discussion, and these are highlighted below.

Because the establishment of a professional relationship with a clinician is a contractual matter, some practitioners might argue that the procedures are selected entirely at the choice of the contracting parties. That is, if the consumer, client, or patient determines that the practitioner is competent enough for his or her purposes (and the practitioner agrees that he or she is competent to provide such services), that should be sufficient. Common examples of such assumptions include the following: A community-organization trained social worker who believes that licensing is a guild process and refuses to obtain a license and is employed by a community agency which has full knowledge of the circumstances; an industrial-organizational psychologist who believes that his or her work with individuals is not clinical service and refuses to obtain a license, and who provides occasional marital "advice" to consultees in the organization; a marriage and family therapist who believes that the licensing examination in his or her profession is unfair and refuses to sit for it, holding himself or herself out as a "mental health advisor" and making it clear that no third-party reimbursement is possible for the services.

However, a key assumption of the process of protecting the public is the notion that in the selection of professionals (be they accountants, psychotherapists, or electricians) the layperson is *not* able to adequately judge whether he or she is being well served. A full discussion of this debate is beyond the scope of this book; for further consideration of this issue as a public policy question, see Faden and Beauchamp (1986). From the perspective of protecting the public, however, the licensing process, however flawed, is justifiable. It is justifiable even though all that it can realistically signify is that an individual is able to demonstrate attainment of minimum levels of knowledge, education, and experience; it by no means guarantees competent or ethical practice. Given the practical, legal, and ethical questions raised, it is difficult to conceive of situations in which a practitioner who claims to deliver competent service is justified in not seeking the appropriate licensure or certification.

SELF-ASSESSMENT OF ONE'S OWN COMPETENCE

We assume the typical practitioner is usually well motivated and does not intentionally practice outside his or her area of professional competence. Nonetheless, it is likely that the cases involving competence heard by licensing boards, ethics committees, professional standards committees, and courts represent only a small fraction of those in which competence is an issue. The circumstances described below illustrate relevant points in this regard.

Example 1. A couple comes to a psychotherapist in private practice requesting sex therapy. The therapist has had no formal coursework in sex therapy, but has read several of the major works in sex therapy and has attended a 2-day workshop on the subject. The therapist feels that he can probably help the couple. Can he consider himself competent to provide the requested service? Should his decision change if he has not read any of the major works in the area but has attended a workshop and has a knowledgeable colleague with whom he talks fairly often? Is he competent to conduct sex therapy?

Example 2. A psychotherapist who has had considerable coursework and supervised experience in family therapy and who views herself as competent in this specialty is approached for treatment by an African-American family. They are concerned about their teenage son and his failure to obey family rules. The therapist lives in an area in which there are few minority families, and this is the first

African-American family that she has worked with. Is she competent to deliver this type of service? Would this judgment change if she has worked with several black families, but this is the first family she has worked with in which the son is receiving kidney dialysis? Is she still competent to deliver services?

The previous examples highlight some of the problems encountered in assessing one's competence. Although we have noted that a key component of competence is knowledge, how much knowledge is enough? Is one class enough? Is a 2-day workshop enough? Is reading a couple of books and talking to peers enough? Second, an important problem is that all clinical problems exist in particular contexts, and the context can dramatically change the requirements for competent service. The major issue here is defining what are general clinical principles that transcend particular contexts, and what are specific "micro-competencies" that are needed to deal effectively with unique client populations or circumstances. It is also important to remember that competence is not a static concept. Rather, it must be evaluated against the changing context of existing knowledge in the field. Thus, it is possible for one's competence to "erode" or "decay" over time. We discuss this further in Chapter 16.

These questions are not easily resolved. No credentialing body can possibly anticipate all possible situations a practitioner is likely to encounter and establish standards accordingly. Yet at the same time, the practitioner will be held responsible for delivering competent services even in the absence of such standards. Although the decision-making process in such cases is of necessity abstract and ill-defined, listed below are some factors that one may find useful to consider in assessing his or her own competence to deal with a particular case. We assume that the practitioner is licensed in the profession for which he or she has been trained.

GUIDELINES FOR ASSESSING ONE'S COMPETENCE

Do Relevant Standards Exist? When deciding whether one is competent to deal with a particular clinical problem, an important consideration relates to whether or not there are established educational or practice guidelines. Standards have been developed for practice within some specialty areas. For instance, the American Association of Sex Educators, Counselors, and Therapists has established training and educational guidelines pertaining to the practice of sex therapy in clinical settings. Guidelines have also been established for hypnotherapists, group therapists, and a number of other specialties.

Such guidelines establish in a general way knowledge and educational standards of practice; however, they cannot anticipate all circumstances that practitioners will encounter. At best, they can increase the probability that practitioners know what to do. Whether they actually do what they know how to do is a matter entirely in the hands of the clinician. Nonetheless, in an area in which such standards exist, the clinician would be wise to obtain the appropriate credentials. A therapist who is considering accepting a client who needs services for which standards exist and who does not meet those standards faces increased responsibility to justify delivering such services.

What about clinical areas in which more than one set of standards exist? That is, although the practitioner may be licensed and thus legally qualified to perform various clinical services, how should he or she deal with the more stringent set of specialty and practice guidelines, such as various forms of board certification? Is the practitioner ethically mandated to obtain all relevant credentials? In making such decisions, the practitioner may want to consider the distinction between mandatory and aspirational ethics described earlier. The mandatory, or floor, requirement would be represented by the lowest level of qualification that would allow a practitioner to perform the service in question. For instance, in performing family therapy, it is mandatory that the practitioner be licensed or certified in a field that includes family therapy in its scope of practice. Would obtaining advanced credentials - for example, board certification such as that offered by the American Board of Family Psychology - represent aspirational ethics, representing the practitioner's ongoing process of growth and development? Or is the practitioner obligated to justify his or her failure to obtain advanced credentials in a field in which he or she wishes to specialize?

Is Your Approach Solidly Grounded in Research or Theory? A key feature that distinguishes mental health practice from religious approaches and faith healing is the emphasis on empirical foundations. Thus, the activities of the mental health professional are assumed to be grounded in the best available theory and research. When this notion is translated into the obligations for the individual provider, it becomes clear that the practitioner is obligated to be familiar with research and theoretical findings in the areas with which he or she deals.

This is somewhat easier said than done, however. Primarily, the reason for this difficulty is that there is a time lag between the point at which a critical mass of practitioners encounter a new problem and the point at which researchers can study the problem, not to speak of developing a body of research that makes clear the optimum treatment of the problem. It is the nature of professional work that new problems are always emerging. The ethical practitioner who consults the literature or knowledgeable colleagues about new problems may be actually on the forefront in certain clinical areas. Thus, the ethical practitioner should both search the literature to find what has gone before and consider helping to create the emerging literature by reporting unusual cases or potential innovations in technique. This topic will be touched upon again in the chapter on clinical research, but it is worth noting that from this perspective the research-and-publication enterprise takes on an ethical dimension.

Assuming that the practitioner is confronting a problem that is not rare or previously unheard of, it is important that each practitioner know where to access the existing data, even if those data were not part of his or her training originally. Thus, having access to professional information sources (particularly peer-reviewed journals) as well as to colleagues with relevant expertise is part of maintaining one's competence in a particular area. This notion adds an ethical dimension to the issue of professional isolation.

Despite access to existing research, it may be that there are contradictory findings existing in the literature. The research literature may contain conflicting recommendations, or no obvious practical implications at all. This is often a problem that frustrated practitioners report when they attempt to derive implications for action from their readings of the scientific reports. This increases the obligation on the practitioner to understand the limitations of empirical research in the mental health sciences and to be able to infer implications for practice from it. For example, a therapist may be persuaded that aversion techniques hold great promise for treating habit disorders. However, reviewing the literature reveals many contradictory studies. Which ones are most relevant? In order to answer this question, the clinician must have (or be able to obtain) information about the appropriateness of the sample (e.g., Was the study conducted with college students or true agoraphobics?), the techniques employed (Was it "real" aversion as practiced in a clinical setting?), and the statistical analyses used (Was the effect big enough to be practically meaningful or statistically significant only because of a large sample size?).

Competence has a legal dimension as well. Licensed practitioners can be held professionally liable for failing to deliver reasonably competent service. This is the basis for the malpractice claim of professional negligence. Legal authorities interpret "competent service" to mean having and using the knowledge and skill ordinarily possessed or employed by a member in good standing of the profession (Keeton, 1984). In the past, conforming to local custom (whether or not this was in keeping with current findings) was held to protect the practitioner from findings of negligence (King, 1986). However, local standards of practice have essentially given way to national standards. It is assumed that practitioners have access to the sources of information that would allow them to stay current with nationally emerging findings.

What Contextual Constraints Apply? Just as clinical problems are always nested in a particular context, so is clinical competence dependent on *its* context. For instance, whether one should be considered capable of handling a particular case has some relationship to other services available to the client. In a small community with only a handful of therapists, the only alternative to accepting a wide range of cases may be to deny treatment to patients (and to commit professional suicide). In more urban settings, the alternative to referring to better-trained specialists (and subspecialists) may be to risk malpractice actions (and professional suicide). The *client's* perception of alternatives is also relevant in this regard. If a therapist believes that the client may not continue with treatment if referred to a specialist, then the option of keeping the client (and perhaps obtaining consultation) becomes more defensible.

It is often the case that practitioners working in an institutional setting are expected to work with all cases assigned to them. In such environments, refusing clients because of self-perceived inability to deal with the presenting problems may be impractical or politically unwise. The practitioner in such cases has an increased responsibility to obtain appropriate inservice training, supervision, or continuing education of some sort to provide the best treatment to the patient.

Are You Emotionally Able to Help the Client? In addition to deficits in skills or knowledge, competence can be diminished in a number of other ways. These include such problems as countertransference, personal preoccupations, transient stress, "engagement" (Beier & Young, 1984) with the client, stereotyping, and the like. These difficulties present technical as well as ethical issues, because recognizing them and overcoming them are part of what it means to be a competent psychotherapist.

For example, the psychotherapist who is recently divorced may be at special risk for introducing distortions into an otherwise competent treatment process; the workaholic therapist who finds himself or herself drowsy or irritable during sessions may be at risk for damaging the working relationship or of missing important therapeutic information. These are simply two examples of ways in which the therapist's difficulties (not necessarily resulting from skill or knowledge deficits) may intrude on competent treatment. Clearly, therapists are human and must learn to recognize their human limitations.

The implications of the foregoing are that therapists should (a) have the ability to monitor themselves accurately, (b) have available consultants to whom they can turn for expert advice and for feedback on their own behavior, (c) have social support networks that can provide "resources" in times of stress and that can help prevent them from becoming "depleted," (d) consider personal therapy (this point may seem obvious, but it is remarkable to us how much resistance there seems to be among mental health practitioners to obtaining personal therapy), (e) have available or consider developing referral sources to whom they can send cases beyond their competence, and (f) have the self-discipline and integrity to limit their practices to those cases with which they can deal competently.

Can the therapist assume that he or she will naturally become aware of impaired functioning? We believe that ordinary human defenses of rationalization and suppression operate all too easily among psychotherapists; thus clinicians should consciously monitor the existence of such conditions. Seeking feedback from trusted associates (and receiving this feedback nondefensively) is of utmost importance in recognizing and correcting potentially disabling conditions.

The incompetent or less-than-competent senior psychologist may be "burned out" (G. Corey, M. S. Corey, & Callanan, 1988) or impaired as a result of psychopathology or substance abuse (Haas & Hall, 1990). Burned-out professionals are characterized by negative attitudes toward themselves, others, work, and life (G. Corey et al., 1988) and may experience a sense of fragmentation stemming from having attempted to do too many professional activities at the same time. Sadly, both burned-out and impaired psychologists sometimes have extreme difficulty becoming aware of their limitations, and forceful confrontation by concerned colleagues is often necessary.

Could You Justify Your Decision to a Group of Your Peers? The "clean, well-lit room" standard can prove very useful in making decisions about one's competence to handle a particular situation. The clinician should be aware of prevailing clinical standards and practices, and if deviating from them, ask himself or herself how that might be justified. Because there is very little scrutiny of the vast majority of treatment decisions made by practitioners, it is easy to become casual and lose sight of appropriate standards, making decisions that are significantly at variance with common practices. This speaks to the importance of maintaining active contacts and involvements in one's professional community. It also speaks to the importance of making decisions with current standards of practice in mind. Clinical practice is so varied that many different approaches are acceptable, but underlying these specific approaches is a set of values (some standards of competence included) to which each mental health profession ascribes. Even when working independently, a therapist would do well to ask himself or herself such questions as whether the decisions being made would be the same if a panel of peers were following him or her around, and whether the clinician would recommend the same course of action to others.

Chapter 4

Privacy, Confidentiality, and Privilege in Psychotherapeutic Communications

The closely linked concepts of privacy, confidentiality, and privilege are crucial components of effective clinical practice. Together they represent the guarantee of trustworthiness and safe-keeping - legal, professional, and moral - that the psychotherapist offers to the client. Although empirical data on this issue are sparse, the available evidence (DeKraii & Sales, 1984; Gomes-Schwartz, Hadley, & Strupp, 1978) points out that trust is essential to effective clinical work. Why is this so? The process of psychotherapy typically requires that a client explore and discuss with the therapist information that may be intimate, sensitive, and often painful for the client to acknowledge even to himself or herself. How can we ask a client to trust us enough to share such information with us, if we cannot insure that it will remain the individual's own information, to be shared with others at his or her own discretion?

With this in mind, it is essential that clients understand the protections granted to them in the clinical context, and it is essential that clinicians understand their ethical obligation to protect the confidentiality of clinical information and their legal obligation to respect privileged communications. Further, it is critical that clients and clinicians also know the limits of confidentiality and privilege rights.

This chapter addresses the nature of the interrelated concepts of privacy, confidentiality, and privilege. It discusses some of the limits to confidentiality that the practitioner is likely to encounter. Finally, summary guidelines will be presented to aid the practitioner in decision making about breaching confidentiality.

PRIVACY

The "right to privacy" is a general philosophical concept embedded in a Western view of human dignity (Caplan, 1982). Basically, the notion that individuals have a right to privacy implies that human autonomy carries with it the privilege of keeping secrets. That is, information about oneself should be one's possession, to be dispensed at one's discretion. Elements of a "right to privacy" can be found in the *Bill of Rights of the United States Constitution*, for example, the right of citizens to be "secure in their persons, house, papers and effects" (Webster, 1956/US Constitution, 4th Amendment), as well as in many other legal precedents. It is a deeply ingrained belief in American society that individuals have a right to keep information about themselves private.

Confidentiality and privilege, to be described below, can be looked at as derivatives of the right to privacy. Both concepts are justified by the general philosophical belief that individuals have a right to keep information about themselves private and by the psychological truth that "exposure" of private information to others can result in psychic damage.

CONFIDENTIALITY

Confidentiality is professional privacy. Information has been shared with another, and that other has the duty to keep private information private. The obligation to uphold confidentiality is a key component of the ethical codes of all mental health professions. For example, the *Ethical Principles of Psychologists and Code of Conduct* (American Psychological Association, 1992) states, "Psychologists have a primary obligation and take reasonable precautions to respect the confidentiality rights of those with whom they work or consult, recognizing that confidentiality may be established by law, institutional rules, or professional or scientific relationships" (§5.02). The psychiatrists' code notes, "Confidentiality is essential to psychiatric treatment" (American Psychiatric Association, 1993, §4.1). Social workers are urged to "respect the privacy of clients and hold in confidence all information obtained in the course of professional service" (NASW, 1993, §II.H.). Marriage and family therapists "have unique confidentiality concerns because the client in a therapeutic relationship may be more than one person. Therapists respect and guard confidences of each individual client" (AAMFT, 1991, §2).

Maintaining client confidences protects more than just the particular client-therapist relationship. It also protects the public trust in the mental health professions more generally. If practitioners are perceived to be "loose-lipped" (e.g., as a result of being heard discussing their clients), clients or prospective clients may be inhibited about discussing sensitive matters.

In addition to the ethical dimension of confidentiality, there are some legal issues that bear mentioning. First, licensing statutes frequently incorporate the profession's ethical standards into their language. This makes the licensed practitioner legally bound to uphold confidentiality. Second, legal precedents regarding what constitutes usual and customary treatment (DeKraii & Sales, 1984) may well put the practitioner who breaches confidentiality at risk even in the absence of a specific statute.

PRIVILEGE

Privileged communications are related to admissions in court, as opposed to confidentiality, which deals with all communications (see Knapp & VandeCreek, 1987). The concept of privilege is a legal rather than an ethical one (Cohen & Mariano, 1982). Specifically, privilege statutes grant patients of certain providers the right to prevent the provider from revealing information in a court proceeding. Such privilege statutes indicate that the state's legislative bodies consider the preservation of the trust relationship between helper and client to be more important than the need of the courts to have access to all information potentially usable as evidence.

One distinction between privilege and confidentiality is that privilege is a legally guaranteed right of the consumer, whereas confidentiality is an ethical obligation of the service provider. It must be noted that privilege can be waived by the client but not by the professional (Schwartz, 1989). That is, the clinician does not have the right to reveal privileged information against the client's wishes (unless ordered to do so by the court); nor does the clinician have the right to maintain that communications are privileged if the client waives privilege.

Privilege is not granted to all mental health professionals. State statutes vary in terms of the classes of practitioners to whom privilege is granted. Clinicians should consult local statutes in order to determine whether client communication is privileged. They should also bear in mind that federal courts have a different view of privilege than do state courts (Knapp & VandeCreek, 1987); there is no specific privilege statute in the Federal Code, and therefore in civil cases federal courts appear to be able to apply state privilege statutes depending on the nature of the case. In criminal cases, privilege is governed by *Federal Rule of Evidence 501*, which requires that privilege be analyzed in the light of reason and experience. Thus, because different federal courts have applied this general rule in different ways, it is important to obtain legal consultation if one is dealing with the release of confidential information in federal courts.

It must also be noted that privilege is not absolute. It may be qualified by state law, as in cases of suspected child abuse. In fact, in any judicial proceeding, judges are the ultimate interpreters of when and how privilege applies, and judges seem to differ in terms of the extent to which they honor privilege. Despite this, it is very important that clinicians not be too hasty in revealing privileged information. They should honor the client's privilege until clearly ordered not to do so by the court (R. L. Schwitzgebel & R. K. Schwitzgebel, 1980).

COMPLICATED
CONFIDENTIALITY SITUATIONS

The existence of ethical mandates and legal rulings still leaves many difficult confidentiality decisions in the hands of the professional. Clearly, protecting confidentiality is important, but it should be kept in mind that confidentiality is not an end in itself; rather, it is a means to the end of effective, responsible, caring treatment of emotional or behavioral distress. In this section we focus on a number of complicated situations in which other demands impinge on the mental health professional that may affect the decision whether to breach or protect confidentiality. This discussion does not include consideration of routine requests for information from other professionals or third-party payors for which the client has voluntarily given permission; such situations do not typically represent an ethical question or dilemma. Circumstances to be considered are as follows:

1. Court subpoenas
2. Duty to warn, protect, or report
3. Requests for information from family members
4. Custody issues
5. Group treatment
6. Uncertainty about "who is the client?"
7. Multiple staff in an agency
8. Professional needs (consultation, teaching, support)

COURT SUBPOENAS

The receipt of a subpoena, despite its official nature, does not mean that the practitioner must immediately release whatever information is requested (this point will be discussed further in the chapter on record keeping). On the other hand, it is obviously unwise to rely on the fact that one has the statutory protection of privilege and therefore refuse to respond to a court order. As noted earlier, regardless of state statutes to the contrary, judges may feel that it is within their power to insist on disclosure of information in particular court cases (Cohen & Mariano, 1982). The judge's authority to find a professional in contempt of court is important to remember in this regard. Also, because the client "owns" the privilege, the decision to waive privilege or insist upon it should include the client's wishes. This fact does not absolve the professional of ethical responsibility to advise the client about the potential risks of disclosure, however. It may also be ethically proper to consider negotiating less damaging alternatives to revealing information in open court.   Options may include holding a private meeting in the judge's chambers or the therapist providing written summary to be released to both attorneys and to the judge.

If the client does not waive privilege, then the prudent course for the professional to follow is to obtain legal consultation (Bennett et al., 1990).   Such issues as the nature of the subpoena, relevant privilege statutes, the desires of the client, and possible negative consequences of revealing the information are relevant, and unless very familiar to the practitioner, would be clarified with legal help.   If the client has an attorney, it is wise to consult with this person as well.

DUTY TO WARN, PROTECT, OR REPORT

Initially crystallized as legal doctrine by the now-famous *Tarasoff* decision (*Tarasoff v. Board of Regents of University of California*, 1976), the duty to protect mandates that when practitioners become aware of a threat of physical harm to an identifiable individual or individuals, they incur a duty to take some action to protect the intended victim from their client.   Although earlier interpretations by many clinicians translated this obligation as a "duty to warn" (Bersoff, 1976), it is more accurate to describe the legal obligation as a "duty to protect" (VandeCreek & Knapp, 1993).   As described in the chapter on paternalism, this latter interpretation (unless superseded by local state court rulings or statutes) gives the practitioner more options in deciding what actions may be taken.

The duty to report is similar to the duty to protect and is based on belief that certain conditions are considered by the state to be so dangerous, either to the public welfare or to specific individuals, that reports of their existence must be made regardless of the potential harm to the treatment process.   The duty to report is, in theory, simpler to discharge than duties to warn or protect, in the sense that the duty is typically discharged by a phone call to the proper authorities.

The most notable example of the duty to report, embodied in the statutes of all 50 states (Butz, 1985; VandeCreek & Knapp,

1993), is the duty to report suspected child abuse (in recent years, roughly 20 states have also passed "adult-abuse" reporting statutes as well). Although this duty is incumbent on any citizen, it has been explicitly extended to cover health-care professionals (as well as teachers and social service workers), in that practitioners are in an extremely good position to detect evidence of possible child abuse. Although substantial numbers of practitioners violate these statutes (Kalichman & Craig, 1991), clinicians who do so place themselves in an extremely vulnerable position. From a legal perspective, the nonreporting clinician has decided to violate the law (presumably in favor of some more valued outcome such as maintaining a productive treatment relationship, or perhaps because of doubts about the usefulness of reporting and the wish to spare the family this difficulty). From an ethical perspective, the nonreporting clinician has decided that continued treatment without reporting is in the best interests of the child and the parent(s), and has thus taken on greater responsibility for insuring that treatment does indeed improve the parent's ability to master his or her acting out. The problem with almost all of the statutes is that they mandate reporting only on suspicion of abuse, and thus the psychotherapist may be reluctant to involve the family in a child abuse investigation only on suspected problems; on the other hand, the therapist is himself or herself liable to prosecution if a district attorney decides that the suspicion should have reached the threshold for reporting (VandeCreek & Knapp, 1993). The prudent clinician will know what the definition of abuse is in the state in which he or she practices (definitions differ), and will have thought through (preferably in advance, and possibly with the client directly) what the steps in reporting should be. For example, it is sometimes recommended that helping parents to report directly is preferable (in terms of their later treatment by the child-protection agency) than having the professional report (VandeCreek & Knapp, 1993).

The human immunodeficiency virus (HIV) creates special legal and ethical challenges. The number of individuals infected with the HIV virus, the spread of this virus, and the devastating effects of AIDS have created ethical dilemmas for clinicians who work with HIV-infected clients. In many respects these dilemmas are similar to those posed by potentially violent or potentially abusive clients.

It is true that any sexually transmitted disease raises the issue of risks to which an unwitting sexual partner is exposed. However, the incurable and fatal nature of HIV infection has brought to the forefront of clinicians' consciousness the dangers faced by the sexual partners of their HIV-positive clients. This realization may force clinicians to consider the ethical issues involved in finding a balance among several different concerns: (a) contending with the presenting issue that brings the client to treatment (often it is *not* the issue of how to insure that they keep partners safe from HIV infection); (b) the maintenance of a productive therapy relationship; (c) improving the client's ability to confront and resolve the problems revealed by their failure to inform the partner or to practice safe sex; and (d) the duty (if any) to protect the well-being of sexual partners ignorant of the risks to which they are exposed.

It is important to note in this regard that a substantial number of HIV-positive individuals do not intend to reveal their serostatus to sexual partners (Kegeles, Catania, & Coates, 1988). An example may illuminate some of the issues. A psychotherapist sees a young woman who has recently discovered that she tests positive for HIV, which she presumably contracted through her intravenous use of drugs. She has one primary sexual partner and several occasional sexual partners. She has not told any of them that she tests positive. In most cases the clinician would be permitted, but not required, to report her condition to her partners, but to do so may seriously impair the quality of the therapeutic relationship. It could be that the partners may be protected but the client may leave treatment prematurely, thus preventing her from resolving whatever psychological conflicts led her to keep this information from them in the first place and possibly endangering other potential sexual partners. Thus, it is probably clinically wiser, at least as a first step, to discuss the issue and help the client see the wisdom of revealing her condition to her partners herself. Current case law does not suggest that the therapist is liable should the woman infect a partner, but case law continually changes.

There could be many variations in the types of situations with which a clinician is confronted in working with an HIV-positive client, and the appropriate course of action may vary (Erickson, 1990). There are a number of factors which must be kept in mind in addition to the general consideration that it is preferable to handle situations within a clinical context and with the client's cooperation. First, a number of states have enacted laws pertaining to HIV infection (Macklin, 1991). Second, standards have been developed by various mental health professional organizations. Such standards, along with state laws, typically leave much to the professional discretion of the clinician.

There are several issues to be addressed with regard to HIV and AIDS. First, the precedents for reporting (to health authorities, at least) that one's patient has an infectious disease is long established in medicine. Second, a substantial proportion of HIV-infected individuals will not reveal to their sexual partners, especially "nonprimary" partners, that they are infected (Knapp & VandeCreek, 1990). There are ambiguities in the situation: In what sense is the sexual partner identifiable to the therapist? Is there a moral obligation either way, absent a legal obligation, to report or to maintain confidentiality? Is there foreseeable harm (the standard established in *Tarasoff*-like decisions)? Knapp and VandeCreek (1990), in an interesting discussion of this problem, suggest that it is incumbent upon therapists who have HIV-positive clients to ascertain how much risk the clients are placing on their partners, as different sexual practices entail differing degrees of risk. Most likely, the therapist will have to face these issues even if the HIV status of the patient is unknown (especially if the patient engages in high-risk behavior and refuses to get tested). Position statements by the American Psychological Association and the American Psychiatric Association place the burden on the therapist, indicating that it is not required - but is also not prohibited - to break confidentiality when danger is imminent. Other sources of information (e.g., Beck, 1982) suggest that openness about the risks the patient is running, and openness about the need to allow the partner to make an informed decision, can actually result in better outcomes (e.g., patient or therapist does disclose, and treatment continues).

REQUESTS FOR INFORMATION
FROM FAMILY MEMBERS

Often, for more or less pressing reasons, members of a client's family will contact the clinician and reveal or request information. Although the most common cases concern parents inquiring about their children's treatment, difficult ethical questions arise for the practitioner whether the confidentiality issue concerns a child or an adult. Each of these circumstances will be described below.

When the Client Is a Child. Does a child have a right to confidentiality? Legally, no. In most cases, the parents, as the legal guardians responsible for the child, have the right to know what is going on in treatment.   In fact, if the parent does not protect the child's well-being, he or she is vulnerable to charges of child neglect. It is important for the practitioner to be sensitive to the parent's legal obligation to know what is going on in treatment, as well as to the parent's emotional concerns for the child.

On the other hand, regardless of the legalities, it may be desirable from a practical or ethical perspective to offer the child the same assurances of confidentiality that would be offered to an adult. Technically, to do this, the parent must waive his or her rights of access to the information. It is obviously much better to obtain this permission before treatment begins, rather than trying to negotiate it in the heat of a crisis. Ideally, both child and parent should know under what circumstances (e.g., life-threatening situations) confidential information will be revealed.

When the Client Is an Adult. Family members often feel that they have a right to know what is going on in treatment with a family member (e.g., "I'm her husband, and she should have no secrets from me"). Although an adult client in individual treatment has rights of confidentiality even with respect to other family members, the situation becomes more complicated when the practitioner is working with a couple or a family and sees the clients together at some times and separately at other times. If a client reveals information in an individual session, should another family member have access to that information? If the family is clearly the "client," then a case could be made that revealing such information would be ethically justified. However, based on assumptions about the principle of confidentiality, a client may assume the confidentiality is extended to individuals, not systems. Thus, he or she could reasonably expect that information shared with the clinician individually is confidential, even if other family members are being seen. There may, of course, be sound reasons for acting on different principles (cf. Karpel, 1980). Practitioners who provide marital or family therapy must have thought through in advance their policies with regard to revealing information to members of the couple/family separately, as well as their policies regarding whether to allow the disclosure of "secret" information to the therapist when other members of the couple/family are not present. Explaining (preferably in writing), negotiating, and obtaining clients' consent to proceed at the outset of treatment are all obviously good practices to follow.

An issue which has been receiving increased attention relates to the question of the confidentiality of an adult who is severely mentally ill and whose family members request information. Various individuals and advocacy groups have complained that clinicians are too stringent in their interpretations of confidentiality rights in families of schizophrenic and other mentally ill adults and share too little information with the family members, who often are the primary caregivers of these individuals (Petrila & Sadoff, 1992).

There are many considerations that must be raised in dealing with whether to reveal information to the family of a mentally ill client. The first relates to the clinician's own attitudes. We are aware of situations in which a clinician has refused to give information to the family of a schizophrenic client, citing confidentiality as the reason, when he did not even bother to ask the client what she wanted to have done. It is important that confidentiality not be used as a smoke screen for personal convenience.

It is our belief that in cases when the family of a mentally ill client requests information, the clinician consults the client, and the client refuses to grant permission, this refusal must ordinarily be honored, even if the refusal is based on some type of delusional thinking. That is, the presence of a mental illness does not necessarily eliminate an individual's civil rights, including the right to confidentiality. The exception to this, in our estimation, is when there is a reason to believe that the client is unable to take care of himself or herself and needs someone to act on his or her behalf. For instance, a psychotic client in the midst of an acute exacerbation of symptoms may need to be involuntarily committed, and it is appropriate to seek the family's assistance in this matter. However, once the crisis is past, normal rules of confidentiality must again apply.

CUSTODY ISSUES

Not infrequently, after marital or family (or even individual) treatment has been delivered, families break up. If a custody battle ensues, one or the other partner may subpoena the practitioner or the treatment records. In such cases the practitioner may have few legal grounds on which to resist a subpoena. Although practitioners may believe that they are protected by privileged-communication statutes, Knapp and VandeCreek (1987) cite several ways in which courts may override patient-therapist privilege when the interests of a child are at stake in a custody dispute. Nonetheless, if pretreatment agreements can be negotiated that prevent one member of the couple from subpoenaing information without the consent of the other member, the clinician may possibly be on firmer ground. Although the pretreatment arrangement is probably not legally binding, it may dissuade parties from seeking the notes from conjoint therapy.

Direction in releasing such information is provided by the AAMFT *Code of Ethics* as it states, "In circumstances where more than one person in a family receives therapy, each such family member who is legally competent to execute a waiver must agree to the waiver. . . . Without such a waiver from each family member legally competent to execute a waiver, a therapist cannot disclose information received from any family member" (AAMFT, 1991, §2.1).

From the ethical point of view, practitioners must do what is in the best interest of the client. But in this case, who is the client? Some practitioners take the position that they will provide no testimony in future divorce or custody actions once they have seen a couple together. Others, who have seen only one member of the couple, may find that it is inappropriate for them to testify without direct experience with the other member of the marital pair. Clearly, the most advantageous position is to negotiate these issues beforehand. It is also important in custody cases to distinguish between the role of expert witness (who may be entitled to give an opinion on the relative fitness of each of the parents) and the role of fact witness (who is restricted to reporting what he or she has observed). The difficulties encountered by therapists who submit to subpoena by one party when they have seen them both, or who agree to testify as evaluators when they have functioned as therapists are detailed elsewhere (cf. Haas, 1993).

GROUP TREATMENT

The practice of group psychotherapy places a unique demand on the clinician. Here, information can be just as sensitive and personal as it is in individual therapy, but other clients who do not share the clinician's obligation to protect confidentiality become privy to the information. The practitioner has an obligation to take whatever steps are possible to safeguard the confidentiality of the information shared in groups. At the very least, the group members' responsibility to keep information confidential should be emphasized during the first session, and this should be reiterated as often as needed (e.g., when new members join the group, or when a member feels vulnerable about something that has been shared). Also, the practitioner might consider making himself or herself available to see a client individually to deal with very sensitive information. In the course of such an individual session, the practitioner could discuss the matter with the client and decide together whether or not it should be shared with other group members. This alternative may be unacceptable to practitioners who hold firmly to the rule that there should be no secrets from other group members, but such practitioners may have an added responsibility to assure confidentiality within the group.

UNCERTAINTY ABOUT
"WHO IS THE CLIENT?"

As will be described in more depth in the chapter on loyalty conflicts, at times it may be unclear who the client is. For instance, if a practitioner is hired by the correctional system to provide psychotherapy for a prison inmate, there are questions regarding what guarantees of confidentiality can be provided to the inmate. Although this will be discussed in more detail in Chapter 8, the preferred solution is to anticipate potential problems and negotiate and agree on solutions before treatment begins.

MULTIPLE STAFF IN AN AGENCY

There may be a difference in the assumptions made by a practitioner and a client concerning information to be shared with other staff members in an agency. The practitioner may assume that the agency grants confidentiality to the client so that the case can be openly discussed with other agency personnel, but not outside the agency. The client may, on the other hand, assume that the practitioner grants confidentiality and will discuss the information with no one else. The various codes of ethics seem to favor the client's point of view. That is, the obligation of confidentiality seems to bind the individual practitioner. However, agency personnel often work as teams, and it is frequently imperative that there be open sharing of information among staff members. Because of this, it may be appropriate to inform the client that information may be shared with other staff members and obtain formal permission to do so. If such permission is not forthcoming, alternative arrangements for treatment, such as referral to another practitioner, may have to be made.

As an example of the sort of problems that may emerge when prior consent is not obtained, consider the following: A therapist has been treating a 42-year-old personality-disordered female, and he discovers that she has begun stealing office supplies and money from staff members' purses and wallets. When confronted with this discovery, she abruptly leaves treatment. Several months later, the therapist discovers that she has applied for treatment at another unit of the agency. He informs the staff there of her previous behavior, and she subsequently files an ethics charge, claiming breach of confidentiality. Although it is unlikely that severe ethical sanctions would result from this behavior, the difficulty could have been prevented by informing the woman of information-sharing practices when she began treatment.

PROFESSIONAL NEEDS
(CONSULTATION, TEACHING, SUPPORT)

Certain threats to confidentiality emerge in the context of practitioners' relations with other professionals, particularly in consultation and teaching situations. In such roles, practitioners may want to use clinical information as examples or illustrations. The use of this information is not necessarily for the benefit of the client; rather, its purpose is to instruct. The ethical principles of various disciplines are ambiguous regarding these situations. They mandate either that the information be disguised so that the client is unidentifiable, or that the client give consent before information is shared. The same would apply to published case illustrations.

For most, if not all, practitioners, the temptation to share clinical information with friends or family members can be overwhelming. At times, the practitioner may be feeling considerable stress and may need to ventilate or seek support. At other times, however, the motivation is simply to gossip or share an interesting story.

The mental health needs of the practitioner are obviously important and need to be sustained. If the practitioner needs the support of a trusted and reliable intimate, he or she should obviously not reveal the identity of any client being discussed. In addition, the practitioner should also assure that the confidant is aware and respectful of the highly sensitive and confidential nature of the information being shared. Such sharing should not be accomplished at the expense of the client's privacy or dignity. Discussions that fall into the latter category are those that serve primarily to entertain the audience, enhance the status of the speaker, or demean the subject of the story. These types of "sharing" would ordinarily be considered gossip.

Gossiping, especially gossiping that would threaten the client's dignity or make the practitioner appear unprofessional, should obviously be avoided. However, as Caruth (1985) has discussed, the motivation to gossip may stem from a need to create distance from the client. Additionally, professional gossip may serve as a means of competing with or establishing superiority over one's colleagues. Consider the following example: A clinician meets the supervisor (another mental health professional) of one of her clients at a party. In the context of a discussion of dissociative disorders, the clinician comments, "I'm working with one of your supervisees, and she's the worst borderline I've ever dealt with." The consequences of such a conversation should be obvious.

GUIDELINES: WHEN TO
BREACH CONFIDENTIALITY

In the course of clinical practice, a professional is certain to face numerous situations in which he or she will have to consider breaching confidentiality. For example, a child reveals that she has been sexually abused, a client shows signs of being suicidal or violent, or a request for information is received from a referring practitioner or family member. In some cases, the appropriate decision may be clear-cut, but others may place significant demands on the clinician's judgment.

Based on the preceding considerations and using the key questions from the flow chart presented in Chapter 2, some guidelines can be generated from its components regarding when it may be appropriate to breach confidentiality.

1. *Does a relevant, professional, legal, or social standard exist?* In this case, the relevant standard is that information obtained in the course of treatment is confidential.
2. *Is there a reason to deviate from the standard?* Keeping in mind that confidentiality is a means to an end, and that perfect confidentiality is practically impossible to guaran-

tee, is there another ethical principle or legal requirement that justifies breaching confidentiality? A request for information from a family member, for instance, may not satisfy this requirement unless competing ethical or legal principles such as welfare of the client are raised. However, the duty to protect or report may constitute such a reason to deviate.

An important facet of dealing with this question is whether or not a solution that does not require breaching confidentiality can be generated. For instance, a practitioner may be satisfied that a potentially suicidal patient's "no-suicide contract" will be adhered to, may have an excellent therapeutic relationship with the patient, and may have been given the preferred means of self-destruction (e.g., pills, knife, gun); in such a case, he or she may be able to avoid the need to contact family members.

3. *Can a primary ethical dimension be specified?* In some cases, only one ethical dimension will be obvious, but frequently such cases present little difficulty, at least from the perspective of determining which course of action is ethically appropriate (*implementing* the appropriate action, of course, may be extremely complicated - see below). In the majority of cases in which there are ethical dilemmas, more than one ethical issue may be at stake. While deciding which ethical dimension is "primary" can be quite subjective, there are certainly occasions when such a determination can be made. Decision making can be simplified in such cases by focusing on the most important ethical issue.

4. *Does the new course of action appear to satisfy the needs/preferences of affected parties?* The principle of autonomy (as well as the aims of much mental health work) suggests that including the wishes of affected parties or "stakeholders" is an important component of ethically appropriate and nonpaternalistic action. While it is not always possible to obtain information about the "real" needs or preferences of stakeholders, educated guesses can be made, consultation can be obtained, and a determination

made as to whether or not the considered action is likely to satisfy affected parties.

5. *Does the course of action present any new ethical problems?* The practitioner should be deliberate in determining this course of action, so that confidentiality is breached to the smallest extent necessary to accomplish the required task. For example, if the police need to be notified about a potentially violent act, they do not need to be told other details about treatment. The act of breaching confidentiality can only be justified if a greater good is accomplished by doing so.

6. *Can the course of action be implemented?* The question of practicality is always a consideration. For instance, if a potentially violent client does not meet the legal requirements for commitment, then commitment is obviously not a practical alternative, and there is no reason to breach confidentiality to get a client committed.

Chapter 5

Informed Consent

Providing the prospective client with the opportunity to give informed consent, implicitly or explicitly, forms a substantial portion of the concerns expressed in the various mental health professions' codes of ethics. However, the reason for this intense focus may not be immediately apparent. What is wrong with, for example, the traditional standard of "doctor knows best"? According to this standard, the patient simply presents himself or herself for treatment, and the doctor tells the patient what to do in order to effect a cure. This approach rests largely on the ethical principle of *beneficence*, which holds that to do good is the ultimate good.

This approach has several shortcomings, however. First, and perhaps most important from an analysis of ethical principles, the "doctor knows best" standard restricts the *autonomy* of the individual. The principle of autonomy holds that it is an ultimate value to treat individuals as free agents. For the doctor to act in such a way as to restrict the patient's autonomy deprives the patient of a crucial aspect of his or her humanness; it may also carry the implication that the individual is incapable of making an intelligent decision about his or her treatment. The obligation to obtain patients' informed consent thus implies a respect for their dignity that rests on fundamental moral assumptions about the nature of the person.

Second, the "doctor knows best" standard is, unfortunately, too easy to abuse. In a number of highly publicized incidents (primarily in medicine), a patient, research subject, or consumer was damaged by treatment (or failure to give an indicated treatment) as a direct result of the provider's or researcher's failure to inform (cf. Faden & Beauchamp, 1986). However, such incidents occur in psychotherapy as well (cf. *Abraham v. Zaslow*, 1970/1974).

Third, the "doctor knows best" standard restricts the chances for the patient to actively participate in his or her own treatment. Especially in mental health work, this is a vital part of successful intervention. The passive patient is perhaps more tolerable in conventional medicine (although this long-held belief is increasingly suspect) but in the psychological domain, simply to tell the patient "sit there and take your medicine" is nonsensical at best, and actually may eliminate a potent avenue of healing at worst.

Thus, the obligation to inform the patient sufficiently that he or she can make a reasoned judgment about accepting or rejecting the proposed treatment is a significant one for the ethical mental health practitioner. It is also a procedure of prudence. Specifically, the therapeutic relationship, and, in fact, any voluntary professional relationship, rests on the consent of the client who initiated it. Moreover, the patient alone has the authority to terminate the relationship without censure. If professionals terminate a treatment relationship without the patient's consent for reasons of their own convenience, they are open to charges of abandonment. Clients have no such obligations, and may unilaterally terminate a professional relationship unless they have legally been committed to treatment.

Despite the clear-cut obligation to inform prospective consumers so that they may make informed decisions, the specifics of providing opportunities for informed consent are far from clear. In part, this is a result of the fact that providing informed consent is both a moral obligation and an exercise of technical skill which will vary depending on the specifics of the case at hand. That is, the manner in which the practitioner provides information and the timing with which he or she provides it can affect whether the information is helpful or harmful. This will be discussed further below.

One often-overlooked benefit of this emphasis on informed consent is that obtaining it may enhance the trust between patient and provider. This issue is effectively discussed, primarily with regard to medicine, by Jonsen et al. (1982). These authors also note that there is a practical reason for obtaining informed consent: increasingly the courts recognize failure to obtain it as evidence of professional negligence.

The idea that one can obtain informed consent from prospective patients implies that they are able to absorb and process information so that they can voluntarily decide whether or not to utilize mental health services. It is true that some clinicians do not consider prospective mental health patients to be capable of autonomous action because of their psychological disturbance (Faden & Beauchamp, 1986). However, because any given prospective patient's degree of disturbance is unknown at the beginning of treatment, the individual should be treated as if he or she has the capacity to act autonomously until there is evidence to the contrary. One simple way to articulate this standard is that the responsible mental health practitioner should attempt to obtain the maximum possible informed consent from patients or clients. Granted, this will not solve all dilemmas (e.g., consider the refusal of a severely mentally ill homeless person to accept referral to a facility), but it is a useful starting point.

This chapter first discusses the nature of informed consent from a legal and psychological perspective. It then deals with considerations in tailoring disclosure to the specific person. Then, the content of the informed consent is covered, followed by a discussion of how to include information. Finally, the chapter addresses the limitations or exceptions to the obligation to provide informed consent.

THE NATURE OF INFORMED CONSENT

Three components are generally considered critical in obtaining informed consent. First, the idea that consent is *informed* implies that enough information has been provided for the potential client to make a reasonable determination whether or not to accept the recommended treatment. Second, the implicit notion underlying informed consent is that it is *voluntary*. Third, the implication in the notion of informed consent is that the consenter is *competent* to make such a determination. Competency refers to the ability to initiate a voluntary action and determine one's choices with at least the degree of autonomy possessed by the average member of one's culture or society.

A corollary of the preceding is that the provider must give information in such a manner that the prospective consumer can understand it. This means that the practitioner should avoid mystifying jargon and should use language comprehensible to the prospective client.

What are the standards for providing such information? One often-used standard has been the "usual and customary professional" standard. That is, the provider is obligated to tell patients only that which the typical provider in his or her community tells patients. This standard has increasingly given way to the "reasonable person" standard, under which the provider must inform the client of any information that might be expected to affect a reasonable person's decision about the recommended procedure. There is, additionally, the less widely used standard called the "subjective understanding" standard (Faden & Beauchamp, 1986). This standard indicates that the practitioner should provide any information that would be material and relevant to the *particular person* to whom the information is being disclosed. This standard, as Faden and Beauchamp discuss, is more difficult to implement in actual practice because it requires that the practitioner know a considerable amount about the prospective patient before treatment begins.

Additional information that is often desired by "reasonable persons" includes the likely duration of treatment, the fact that treatment is voluntary, and the general obligations one expects from patients (e.g., how much notice to give on cancelling appointments, permissibility of home telephone calls, charges for telephone consultations and report writing, if any, etc.). In addition, it is appropriate to offer information about the qualifications of the provider.

In determining what to include as part of an informed consent statement, the practitioner also needs to consider the potential of creating a self-fulfilling prophecy. For instance, to inform a client that some people find psychotherapy stigmatizing may induce the client to respond to people in a more reserved or suspicious manner and, thus, affect the way the client is responded to by others.

By the same token, it could be argued that providing information about positive benefits that the treatment has produced will motivate clients' participation. However, although this at times may be a useful clinical strategy, it is hoped that the client already believes (at least to a limited extent) that treatment may be helpful. The line between discussing the benefits of treatment and guaranteeing a particular outcome should be noted. Inclusion of a specific projected outcome in an informed consent statement could be viewed as a contractual obligation and increase the liability risk of the practitioner (Kenneth Pope, personal communication, 1983). On the other hand, the work of Kahneman and Tversky (1981, 1984) suggests that informing clients about the *benefits* to be obtained from the proposed procedures often is superior to providing the same information couched in "harms to be avoided" when eliciting their consent. Faden and Beauchamp (1986) discuss this issue further; we mention it here to alert the practitioner to consider that the same information can be presented in a variety of ways.

TAILORING DISCLOSURE
TO THE SPECIFIC PERSON

The reality of providing information to patients so that they may make informed decisions is relatively complex. A few examples will illustrate the problem. When one asks what information will be relevant to which consumer with which problem, the actual consent disclosure becomes much more problematic. Does the single retiree who is presenting with problems of depression want to know that you are obligated to report him if he abuses his child (which he doesn't have)? Does the acutely psychotic patient want to know that one of the risks of therapy is that other people may find it a sign of poor adjustment? Clearly, certain information is not relevant to certain individuals. On the other hand, it may be highly relevant to inform a prospective client that his or her insurance company will be asking for information about the diagnosis before deciding whether or not to reimburse. Thus, it is often difficult to determine in advance what information will be needed by a particular client. It is probably better, on balance, to give too much information than too little.

INFORMATION TO INCLUDE IN DISCLOSURE

There is both a content dimension to the task of obtaining informed consent and a process dimension. The content consists of essential information needed by the prospective client in order to enable him or her to make an informed decision. We present what we consider to be the seven minimum domains of information below:

1. *The Risks and Benefits of Treatment.* Depending on the setting in which one practices, risks could include the embarrassment of having other people know that one is in therapy, the stirring up of unpleasant memories, the concern that others may think one is mentally unstable, and the difficulties of obtaining later employment (particularly relevant to inpatient settings). The benefits of treatment typically include more comfortable functioning in social, work, and family settings; decreased negative emotionality; less self-defeating behavior; improved ability to realize life goals; and more satisfying relationships.

2. *Logistics of Treatment.* Typically this information might include how long sessions last (e.g., 50-minute "hours"), how long treatment lasts (e.g., weekly for several months, twice-weekly for several years, etc.), the cost of sessions, the cost of additional services such as telephone contact, letter writing on behalf of the client, testing and test interpretation, types of records kept, billing practices, and policies regarding insurance reimbursement.

3. *Qualifications of the Provider.* Ordinarily this includes highest degree obtained; provider's specialty (e.g., psychology, social work, psychiatry, marriage and family

therapy); board certifications, if any; additional specialty, if any (e.g., hypnosis, family therapy, gestalt, biofeedback); particular disorders or issues emphasized in practice (e.g., divorce, sexual dysfunction, substance abuse); and training and experience in the kind of service being sought by this client (if not covered in the previous items).

4. *Risks and Benefits of Alternatives to Treatment.* In addition to describing what treatment might help to accomplish and what risks it might entail, it may be important to provide parallel information regarding the alternatives to treatment. If there are well-accepted alternatives to the type of treatment one offers, these should be mentioned to the prospective client. If the only alternative to the treatment one offers is no treatment, then the risks of allowing the condition to remain untreated should be explained. Typically, these risks include risk that the condition will simply persist if left untreated, risk that the condition will worsen, and risk that it will become less amenable to treatment over time.

An interesting derivative question is whether the provider is obligated to disclose the risks and benefits of treatments of which he or she disapproves (cf. Jonsen et al., 1982). From an ethical point of view, the practitioner is *permitted* but not *obligated* to disclose such information. However, from a technical or clinical point of view, the practitioner may prefer to disclose such information as a means of more strongly recommending the treatment of choice.

5. *Clarity Regarding Technique.* In the past it was common to remind therapists to obtain informed consent about any "unusual" methods they employed or unusual policies they followed. However, because treatment is so variable across settings and across providers, the definition of "unusual" depends heavily on one's viewpoint. Therefore, therapists should provide as much clarity as they think is necessary regarding their techniques. For example, some therapists use homework assignments, some use concurrent group therapy, some require certain tests, some routinely

schedule family sessions, some routinely make tape recordings of sessions, and so forth.

6. *Emergency Procedures.* The therapist should have a backup or emergency service, and these arrangements should be described. If there is no such service and the therapist has particular recommendations for clients who need after-hours contact, these policies should be described. For example, does the therapist take "crisis" calls at home after hours? Alternatively, does the therapist not publish his or her phone number and instead refer clients to the crisis line of the local community mental health center? It should be noted that use of a covering or backup therapist is likely to compromise confidentiality, as the covering therapist must be given enough information about the case to cover effectively.

7. *Confidentiality and Its Limits.* Although it is commonly expected by prospective clients that confidentiality will be upheld (McGuire, Toal, & Blau, 1985; Rubanowitz, 1987), it is helpful to remind clients both that information they provide will be held confidential and that there are certain limits to this protection. As noted earlier, it is not technically required that therapists inform their clients about the possibility that they will be obliged to breach confidentiality in cases of potential harm to self or others; however, it is wise to mention the duty to protect issue at the outset. Including this information reduces the chance that the client will accuse the therapist of entrapment after the client has revealed information that signals dangerousness. Similar suggestions can be made regarding reporting laws for cases of child abuse, incest, spouse abuse, the planning of crimes, and suicide risk.

HOW TO INCLUDE INFORMATION

Because many patients are eager to "get on" with the discussion of their chief complaint, some practitioners have raised the question of whether it unnecessarily delays treatment (and would therefore be ethically undesirable) to provide the necessary information about treatment and obtain informed consent at the outset. In an interesting recent ethics case involving a mental health professional who failed to disclose his fees to a client, the clinician offered the defense that "therapy had not really begun" because this particular therapist considered the first three to five sessions to be "evaluation" and not "treatment." Needless to say, the client (now ex-client and complainant) prevailed and the therapist was disciplined.

With the most recent revisions of the major mental health professions' ethics codes, this issue of timing is now moot; each one specifies the professional's obligation to inform users of their services at the outset of all relevant information. The psychologists' ethics code (American Psychological Association, 1992) mandates that "Psychologists discuss with clients or patients as early as is feasible in the therapeutic relationship appropriate issues, such as the nature and anticipated course of therapy, fees, and confidentiality" (§4.01a). The psychiatrists' code of ethics (American Psychiatric Association, 1993) indicates that "Psychiatric services, like all medical services, are dispensed in the context of a contractual arrangement between the patient and the treating physician. The provisions of the contractual arrangement, which are binding on the physician as well as on the patient, should be explicitly established" (§2.5). Social workers "should provide clients with accurate and complete information regarding the extent and nature of the services available to them" (NASW, 1993, §II.F.6.). The marriage and family therapists' code (AAMFT, 1991) is less explicit but indirectly supports the need to inform clients and allow them to make their own decisions.

WRITTEN INFORMED CONSENT

Despite the need for full disclosure and informed consent, there is an element of beneficence in the wish to delay treatment of a distressed individual as little as possible. One possible resolution to the problem is to provide written informed consent statements to prospective patients so that they may be digested before the session begins, and less-pressing questions can be dealt with later. This approach too has its advantages and drawbacks. As an advantage, it saves the practitioner the time needed to detail the many possible risks and benefits of treatment, and it also removes some of the more difficult issues from immediate presentation. As a disadvantage, it does not allow the practitioner to assess carefully whether the patient indeed comprehends the proposed treatment. Written promises are also frequently treated as evidence of contractual liability, so such statements must be prepared with extra care (this may be an advantage). Nonetheless, the written "patient information statement" is rapidly becoming the standard of practice (Bennett et al., 1990). Although these authors do not specifically recommend written informed consent statements, they do recommend that if written statements are *not* used, that documentation of the clinician's obtaining informed consent be included in the record). A sample disclosure form developed and used by one of the authors (LJH) in a general outpatient psychology practice is included with the present volume as Appendix E (pp. 259-260). It is offered in the hope that others may use and improve upon it; in the interests of fully informing the reader of the risks and benefits, it should be clear that the responsibility for adapting the statement to one's own state laws, practice environment, and patient population is entirely the user's, not the author's. Older published patient information and treatment contract forms can be found in L. Everstine et al. (1980) and Hare-Mustin et al. (1979).

Written information statements have several advantages: The information can be presented comprehensively, it can be written clearly (editorial consultation may be helpful in this area), and it allows the client to absorb the information at his or her own rate. In addition, written information is consistent across clients, and can be given to patients at the beginning of therapy without interfering unduly with the establishment of the working relationship. Further, written informed consent statements leave a record that one has at least offered certain facts for the client's consideration (whether or not the client absorbs those facts is another story). Finally the provision of an informed consent statement can serve in part to establish an atmosphere of openness about one's services. Of course, it is also possible to send the message that one is legalistically defensive about one's practice. However, with consultation from knowledgeable colleagues and possibly even provisional documents offered to clients for their feedback, the written informed consent statement can be refined so that it sends the message that one is willing to be clear with clients about their rights.

VERBAL INFORMED CONSENT

In addition to making available a written statement of information for prospective clients, informed consent should also be obtained verbally. Verbal informed consent allows the careful assessment of the individual's comprehension of the issues, allows for the providing of information specific to the client's circumstances, and permits the communication of positive affect (such as caring, consideration, kindness, affirmation of the client's independence, respect) that the written format does not permit.

Verbal informed consent can be obtained both "proactively" and "reactively." By proactively obtaining verbal informed consent it is meant that providers should, some time after giving the written document to clients, check to see if the material has been read and understood. The written document may trigger questions which the therapist can then answer. Reactively obtaining verbal informed consent means that the therapist assumes that the client will ask questions if he or she is unclear about an aspect of treatment, and is ready to respond to such questions. The nature of the questions triggered by various events in therapy cannot be predicted, although they usually touch on issues that should have already been presented in the early phases. Of course, one must first establish a climate in which clients feel free to ask such questions. It is remarkable how often clients feel intimidated by their therapists and do not feel such freedom (cf. Dimatteo & Hendricks, 1982).

THE INFORMED CONSENT ATTITUDE

Implicit in the foregoing is the notion that informed consent can be obtained in either a defensive, legalistic manner or in an open, trust-building way. Much of this contextual information is sent nonverbally, and much of it depends on the therapist's level of comfort with his or her practices. The informed consent procedure can be considered as a specific example of a person-environment interaction; the therapist has several parts to play in establishing the appropriate environment. First and foremost, the therapist must be fair with the client without being discouraging about the realities of treatment outcome. On the other hand, the clinician must be optimistic and validate the client's faith in the process without overselling the treatment. No hard-and-fast rules are possible in this regard. A judgment about the client's level of optimism/pessimism, one's own mastery or lack of mastery of the techniques, and the difficulty of the problem at hand all contribute to a contextual judgment of what to say and how to say it. Nonetheless it is hard to imagine "losing therapeutic ground" by treating clients as if they are potential collaborators in their own treatment. Indeed, that is the ultimate goal of much psychological therapy. Informed consent increases the likelihood that clients can challenge what their therapists offer them, and this in turn makes it important to be comfortable with what one does. Indeed, the question of the boundary between appropriate curiosity about aspects of treatment and resistance to such treatment is always a clinical issue to be resolved. Therapists, too, need to resolve the question of when they are simply being withholding because they feel restricted in their practice and when they are intuitively picking up some defensive purpose to the repeated questions raised by clients.

The conventional view of informed consent procedures suggests that all issues be spelled out at the beginning of treatment; however, this may be clinically unrealistic, because it would leave little time for actual clinical work if carried to its logical extreme. Thus it may be more useful to consider the obtaining of informed consent as a process, perhaps beginning with more general and global descriptions of the elements of treatment and later progressing to specific descriptions of specific procedures as needed.

LIMITATIONS TO INFORMED CONSENT

Although the paradigm case for providing information to prospective consumers is that the consumer is an independent, autonomous, competent adult, in reality many other conditions apply. These conditions can compromise any of the aforementioned characteristics. For example, the person may not be considered competent by reason of disabling mental status or of youth; the person may not be in the position to make an informed judgment because of the time pressures or emergency nature of the situation; the person may not be able to consent because of legal constraints; or consent may be limited because of judgment by the professional that the risks of harming the patient through disclosure outweigh the benefits to be gained by involving the patient in a participatory decision. Each of these will be considered in turn below.

YOUTH

The legal age for competence to consent (to such things as contracts and marriages as well as mental health treatment) varies somewhat from state to state and situation to situation, but is typically around age 16 (Plotkin, 1981). This age marker is simply a "proxy" for other characteristics that are assumed to change with age. These include the ability to weigh the consequences of a present course of action for one's future well-being. In the obvious case - that is, a child who is clearly unable to understand the nature of treatment but who obviously needs it - one finds "substituted consent." That is, the responsible party, usually a parent or guardian, consents for the minor. Many authors (e.g., Schetky & Cavanaugh, 1982) note that either parent's consent suffices when the parents are married. However, when divorce has occurred, clinicians must ascertain who has legal custody and obtain consent from that parent. In cases of joint custody, it is prudent to obtain consent from both parents. If legal guardianship resides elsewhere, that person or agency must give consent.

From a clinical standpoint, it is wise to attempt to maximize the child's understanding of the proposed treatment. In the research arena, this is known as obtaining minors' *assent.* As Melton (1981), Holder (1985), and others point out, involving children in treatment decisions improves treatment outcome. Weithorn (1983) cites several studies that have shown, in addition, that the process of involving a child in health-related decision making contributes to an increased sense of personal responsibility for health care. However, from an ethical point of view, involving the child is aspirational rather than mandatory, and from a legal point of view it is usually superfluous. The converse - failure to obtain parental permission - may engender legal and practical, as well as ethical, problems, however. As Schetkey and Cavanaugh (1982) point out, such failure can expose the practitioner to a legal risk of assault (unwanted "touching") if challenged by an aggrieved parent, and may also result in disputes over payment of the bill. As the child enters middle to late adolescence, however, the issue becomes more confusing.

Gaylin (1982) has usefully discriminated between the child's ability to independently *consent* to treatment versus the child's ability to independently *refuse* treatment. Gaylin suggests that the practitioner should give greater weight to the child's willingness to accept treatment in the face of parental disapproval, and somewhat less weight to the child's ability to independently refuse treatment in the face of parental interest in continuing or initiating it. When examining these concepts, it becomes clear that one underlying dimension is the question of the person's judgments about short-term benefits versus long-term costs and benefits. This analysis of the situation suggests that the youngster who is willing to undergo short-term "costs" (e.g., treatment) in the interest of long-term benefits should be taken seriously; however, if the youngster seems to prefer short-term "benefits" (e.g., avoidance of treatment) regardless of long-term "costs" of such a course of action, perhaps more effort should be made to recruit him or her into treatment.

DIMINISHED CAPACITY

In the case of psychotic, retarded, or demented individuals who lack the capacity to give competent informed consent, the concept of "substituted consent" can supplement or replace issues of obtaining informed consent from the patient himself or herself. When it is clear that an individual does not have the capacity to rationally weigh the costs and benefits of treatment, a third party who may be assumed to have the patient's interests at stake can be consulted. It may be the case that no such third party exists, and in such cases the practitioner should turn to an informed party of peers or laypersons. Even in cases of substituted consent, however, it is useful to at least provide the individual an opportunity to assent to the proposed treatment.

EMERGENCIES

True life-threatening emergencies in mental health practice are fortunately rather rare. Typically it is possible to provide the prospective patient with at least a brief description of what is proposed without unduly delaying treatment or causing damage. This is in contrast to the medical situation, in which delay of even a few minutes may be dangerous or in which the patient may present in an unconscious state. Nonetheless it occasionally does occur that patients present with acute mental health emergencies. What are such emergencies? A primary one concerns the suicidal patient. Such individuals are in need of immediate psychological intervention and are probably more concerned about their continued survival than about the long-term costs and benefits of entering treatment.

A second situation that makes it difficult to provide informed consent, at least initially, is that in which a psychotic episode is occurring. Individuals in psychotic states cannot usually be considered competent to provide informed consent. Thus if the situation is one in which time makes a difference, treatment may reasonably be started without obtaining informed consent. If there is more time available, patients' guardians, relatives, or "substituted consent providers" should be contacted. In such cases it is usually permissible to use one's professional judgment to initiate treatment and to delay providing information relevant to informed consent until such time as it may be useful to the patient. Notice that once again the principles of autonomy and beneficence are in conflict, with beneficence winning out.

LEGAL CONSTRAINTS

In certain cases the patient's participation in treatment is nonvoluntary. Such cases include court-ordered treatment (in which case it might reasonably be argued that the "patient" is the court, at least as much as is the individual sitting in the consulting room). Other such cases include those in which a spouse has threatened consequences such as divorce if the person does not seek treatment. These cases are somewhat more difficult if they raise questions about the voluntariness of the consent obtained. As in the preceding case, this raises the question of "Who is the client?" Particularly in cases in which the identified client appears to be feeling coerced, the clinician must carefully evaluate whether the party insisting on treatment should be included in the negotiation of the treatment contract. This may prevent later difficulties if the insistent party is dissatisfied with the progress of therapy. However, even in the absence of clear indications of coercion, the therapist should be especially sensitive to the client's treatment options. If the client cannot be voluntarily involved in the choice of treatment directions (even if he or she might not have chosen to be in treatment), then termination should be considered. The ethical codes of almost all the mental health professions mandate terminating a nonproductive professional relationship, and this policy is consistent with such a mandate.

PROFESSIONAL JUDGMENT

Providers or practitioners may use their professional judgment when it appears that providing informed consent will damage the patient in some way, or in cases in which there is some theoretical rationale for withholding information. It is useful to remember that the provision of informed consent is a means to an end; it is not an end in itself. The end is to emphasize the autonomy and dignity of the individual. This can be done through other means if providing informed consent would potentially harm the treatment relationship or drive the person from suitable treatment. These kinds of cases invoke the conflicting principle of beneficence in contrast to the principle of autonomy.

Hypnotic techniques, especially in Ericksonian therapy, bear on this issue, as do some attempts to enhance transference. More recently, paradoxical therapy has also become a focus of concern. Paradox is most clearly defined by Rohrbaugh (1982) as instructing the client to intensify or enact situations that were described by the client as undesirable. In other words, the therapist is directing the client to do something which the therapist does not actually believe the client should do. Examples of paradoxical suggestions include indicating to clients that they "become more depressed" or suggesting that clients intensify a particular symptom at a particular time. Should the therapist inform the client that actually the therapist is giving these instructions so that the client can get rid of the symptom in question? Many paradoxical therapists argue that revealing the fact that an instruction is intended to be paradoxical renders it useless.

For example, it is not uncommon for therapists who give "symptom prescriptions" as between-session assignments to be asked for the rationale behind this. Answering, "If you don't do this, I'll be forced to refer you" without any additional explanation is unnecessarily harsh (although actually recommended by some advocates). Instead, the therapist could indicate that in his or her best judgment, this technique may prove helpful, and ask the client to try it as an "experiment." It should be noted in passing that there is no empirical support for the idea that informing patients about paradoxical methods reduces their effectiveness. For example, Hills, Gruszkos, and Strong (1985), found that outcomes for clients who were and were not informed about paradoxical techniques did not differ after 30 days. Similarly, Hunsley (1988) argues that providing a rationale does not reduce the usefulness of paradox any more than a rationale for any other intervention reduces its usefulness. Other studies (e.g., Ascher & Turner, 1980) also confirm the notion that paradox "works" even if it is explained. Thus there would appear to be little justification for failing to inform clients that one's directives and suggestions are, even if they appear contrary, designed to improve the client's well-being.

Psychotherapists who use psychoanalytic methods also seem to have trouble reconciling these principles. Such therapists argue that revealing too much about the technique to the patient can contribute to resistance and can interfere with effective treatment.

At the minimum it is clear that providing information is not a dichotomous task. One can certainly provide much essential information without going into technical detail about the nature of one's procedures. It certainly seems reasonable to inform patients that (a) treatment is voluntary, (b) techniques that may not always be of obvious relevance will be employed, and (c) they have the right to ask questions at any time. It seems to us that these concepts could be presented to clients without unduly compromising the therapist's effectiveness.

SUMMARY: GUIDELINES FOR PROVIDING INFORMED CONSENT

The following are practical guidelines for providing the opportunity for informed consent.

1. Assume that the person is competent to give informed consent unless there is clear evidence to the contrary.
2. Put yourself in the patient's place; what information would *you* desire?
3. Use clinical judgment in providing the details of the proposed treatment: How much information can the person absorb? Consider that information overload can prevent the obtaining of informed consent perhaps as much as underdisclosure.
4. If in doubt, inform the person anyway. It is always better to have provided sufficient information than to be accused later of having denied the patient the opportunity to decide for himself or herself.
5. In a conflict between autonomy and beneficence, beneficence is usually given greater weight. However, where conflict exists it is generally wise to seek additional consultation from knowledgeable colleagues or to seek creative technical solutions to the conflict.
6. Put the standard information in writing, give the client a copy of the statement (and keep a signed copy), and have respected colleagues review your statement.

Chapter 6

Dual Relationships:
Avoiding Exploitation
and Maintaining
Appropriate Boundaries

Mental health practitioners occupy many roles in addition to those of psychotherapist, consultant, or evaluator. They are neighbors, friends, relatives, employers, employees, and so on. Typically these roles do not conflict. But increasingly, as the size of the community in which one practices decreases, or as the group with which one practices overlaps more and more with one's other social groups, practitioners run the risk of having additional role relationships with their patients or clients. Many of these "dual relationships" do not raise ethical questions. For example, one's client may also be one's neighbor, and one may encounter this person at neighborhood association meetings or while working in one's yard. Aside from some possible momentary embarrassment and fleeting questions about how best to manage the interaction, this sort of dual relationship is not necessarily ethically problematic. Other dual relationships are more difficult. From an ethical and perhaps a technical standpoint as well, the roles of therapist and lover, therapist and employee, therapist and relative, therapist and instructor, or therapist and supervisor are not compatible. This chapter is focused on the dangers inherent in such dual relationships and offers in addition some guidelines for maintaining one's ethical equilibrium.

Example 1. A male therapist is working with a female client. He has begun a practice of walking her to her car after their sessions, ostensibly to make sure she's safe. Then he begins scheduling her as his last client of the evening. One night, he asks her to have a drink with him, telling her that it would be therapeutic for her to associate with a decent man, as opposed to the losers with whom she usually spends her time. The client is flattered by all of the attention being showered upon her by a man for whom she has great respect, and she goes along with him. One thing leads to another, until eventually they end up in bed. The therapist tells her that sex with him would be good for her psychologically, because he is the type of man she should be associating with; again, she is unquestioning in her trust of the therapist. As the relationships progress, the client begins writing the therapist love letters and calling him at home, and the frequency of such contacts increases to a point where the therapist's wife begins to ask questions. Finally, the therapist tells the client that she is not amenable to treatment and that she will never change, and he abruptly terminates her (from both relationships).

Example 2. A therapist is the coach of her 10-year-old daughter's volleyball team. One of the girls on the team is having a terrible time controlling her anxiety, and her performance during games is inhibited because she is so tense. The therapist discusses the problem with the girl's parents and suggests that they make an appointment to bring the girl in for desensitization therapy. Unfortunately, the girl's anxiety does not improve with treatment; in fact, she gets worse. She tells her parents that she dreads going to practice because she is afraid that she will disappoint her therapist/coach. Her attendance at practices and games becomes more and more sporadic, and she finally drops off the team.

Example 3. Over the course of therapy, a therapist who is treating a couple begins to develop a fondness for them, and they for him. The couple invites the therapist and his wife to a party, and his wife also develops a fondness for the couple. The two couples spend increasing amounts of time together, while the therapist continues to work with them. At a later party, the couple begins to quarrel and attempts to involve the therapist.

Though different in many ways, these examples represent several of the countless instances of problematic dual relationships that can develop. Whereas the term "multiple relationships" has seen increased use in the past years and has become the term used in the *Ethical Principles of Psychologists and Code of Conduct* (American Psychological Association, 1992), we have opted to continue using the term "dual relationships" to describe this particular sort of ethical problem. This is because, although it is true that a practitioner and a consumer of services can be involved in more than two relationships, it is easier to assess the problematic nature of relationships and to evaluate the relevant ethical issues if they are considered two at a time (e.g., a therapist-client relationship combined with a romantic relationship or a consultant-consultee relationship combined with a financial relationship).

As noted previously, many dual relationships do not raise ethical questions, though others are more problematic. The affective and clinical aspects of certain dual relationships have been addressed in depth elsewhere (e.g., Goldberg, 1977; Roy & Freeman, 1976); this chapter will discuss a number of the practical and ethical aspects of dual relationships. We will first discuss general problems that arise when a therapist and a client maintain a dual relationship. Then, some aspects of dual relationships particularly relevant to clinical practice will be described. Finally, we will present guidelines for avoiding potentially problematic dual relationships and maintaining one's ethical equilibrium.

WHEN AND WHY ARE
DUAL RELATIONSHIPS BAD?

Because we are all human beings, it is impossible for us to avoid dual relationships completely. Dual relationships are made almost inevitable by the fact that we all exist in social worlds and interact with people in numerous contexts. The likelihood of encountering a client outside the therapeutic setting is substantial, and it increases with the years a professional has been in practice. In fact, some extra-therapy relationships are a vital source of referrals, and it would raise other ethical questions to refuse to offer services to persons with whom one had other contacts.

The smaller the community, the greater are the chances that dual relationships will develop, until at some point they become a virtual certainty. For instance, a social worker of our acquaintance was asked to conduct family therapy with the family of his own brother - there were simply no other available family therapists (or other types of mental health professionals, for that matter) in the small town in which he practiced. In recent years, increasing attention has been paid to the special problems of dual relationships encountered in rural communities (Horst, 1989; Jennings, 1992; Stockman, 1990). It is important to keep in mind that dual relationships are not inherently unethical. No code of ethical standards for the major mental health professions prohibits all dual relationships, although each stresses the obligation of the ethical professional to be aware of the potential harm that could be caused by dual relationships. There also seems to be an increased awareness that dual relationships cannot be avoided completely. For instance, the AAMFT *Code of Ethics* (1991) states, "Therapists, therefore, make every effort to avoid dual relationships with clients that could impair professional judgment or increase the risk of exploitation. When a dual relationship cannot be avoided, therapists take appropriate professional precautions to ensure judgment is not impaired and no exploitation occurs. Examples of such dual relationships include, but are not limited to, business or close personal relationships with clients. Sexual intimacy with clients is prohibited. Sexual intimacy with former clients for two years following the termination of therapy is prohibited" (§1.2).

The *Ethical Principles of Psychologists and Code of Conduct* (American Psychological Association, 1992) states, "In many communities and situations, it may not be feasible or reasonable for psychologists to avoid social or other nonprofessional contacts with persons such as patients, clients, students, supervisees, or research participants. Psychologists must always be sensitive to the potential harmful effects of other contacts on their work and on those persons with whom they deal. A psychologist refrains from entering into or promising another personal, scientific, professional, financial, or other relationship with such persons if it appears likely that such a relationship reasonably might impair the psychologist's objectivity or otherwise interfere with the psychologist's effectively performing his or her functions as a psychologist, or might harm or exploit the other party" (§1.17a).

According to the NASW Code of Ethics (1993), "The social worker should not condone or engage in any dual or multiple relationships with clients or former clients in which there is a risk of exploitation of or potential harm to the client. The social worker is responsible for setting clear, appropriate, and culturally sensitive boundaries" (§II.F.4.). While not specifically using the term "dual relationships," the Principles of Medical Ethics With Annotations Especially Applicable to Psychiatry (American Psychiatric Association, 1993) raises related issues that are of ethical concern. For instance, it states, "The psychiatrist should diligently guard against exploiting information furnished by the patient and should not use the unique position of power afforded him/her by the psychotherapeutic situation to influence the patient in any way not directly relevant to the treatment goals" (§2.2).

The preceding statements highlight some of the potential problems that can occur if a therapist maintains a dual relationship with a client. Listed below are two specific concerns:

1. *Dual relationships may exploit the client.* The therapeutic relationship involves an asymmetry of power; the therapist discloses little and comes to know the person at his or her most vulnerable point. Because of this asymmetry, it is doubtful whether the client could distinguish between times when the therapist is acting as a therapist and when he or she is acting as a friend, colleague, or the like. There are real questions as to whether a client could make a truly autonomous decision in the face of persuasion by the therapist. If the therapist suggested, for instance, that the client participate in a business venture, would the client be able to distinguish the therapist as a good clini-

cian from the therapist as a bad businessperson. Would the client be able to refuse a joint enterprise without wondering whether the treatment upon which he or she had come to depend might be jeopardized?

2. *Dual relationships may affect the therapist's ability to make appropriate clinical decisions.* If a practitioner maintains a friendship or other nonclinical relationship with a client, this may make it difficult to confront that client about inappropriate behavior; it may affect the type of recommendations that the clinician would make about the client, and so on. It may be hard, for example, to tell a client with whom you maintain a social relationship that you can understand why his children wish to live with their mother (his ex-wife), or that you see no clinically justifiable reason why he should not have to serve a jail sentence for a crime he has committed.

When dual relationships are involved, it becomes significantly more difficult for a clinician to be certain about his or her motives, a judgment which is difficult under the best circumstances. Given the human ability to rationalize, it is extremely easy to mask the real reason that a particular step is being taken behind a motive that sounds clinically justifiable. The practitioner should always be sensitive to this potential.

In summary, dual relationships cannot be avoided completely and are not inherently unethical. However, they provide fertile ground for the development of problematic situations and, therefore, caution is in order. Certain dual relationships, such as those involving sex with a current client, are always unethical, however. In the next section, some dual relationship situations that present special problems for the clinician are discussed.

CLINICALLY RELEVANT
DUAL RELATIONSHIPS

Although the number of potential dual relationships is quite large, a smaller set merits special attention and will be described separately. These include accepting friends or acquaintances as clients, becoming friends with clients, receiving gifts, and engaging in sexual relationships with current or former clients.

ACCEPTING FRIENDS OR ACQUAINTANCES AS CLIENTS

If a therapist were to decide to avoid dual relationships completely, then he or she would refuse to accept anyone as a client with whom there had been any previous nonclinical contact of any sort, and would even refuse to accept anyone with whom he or she shared common friends, or anyone with whom social contact might be a potential in the future. Few independently practicing therapists, however, have such an unlimited referral pool (or such clairvoyance) that they could be so restrictive, although adopting this stance would eliminate a number of potential problems. Rather, many (if not most) clinicians who are not affiliated with agencies take considerable advantage of referrals made by friends, acquaintances, and other individuals known in social contexts. In accepting clients from these sources, special care must be taken to insure that the client has the same autonomy of decision making that he or she would have if the referral were from another source. This is because of the kinds of social obligations unique to this type of referral.

Consider the following possible client reaction: "I think this therapist is incompetent, but Brad and Susan like him, so if I say anything, I'm offending my friends." Or: "If I tell my therapist I don't want any more counseling, I'm going to feel uncomfortable seeing her at the party next week."

The therapist must also examine the limits that the dual relationship will place on his or her response alternatives. If the therapist knows, for instance, that confronting the client will make him or her angry and that the client will likely react by making negative statements about the therapist to mutual friends, there might be a temptation to "pull one's punches" in nontherapeutic ways.

While not specifically an ethical concern, the therapist might be wise also to consider what practical limitations will be placed on his or her social life if an individual is accepted as a client. Therapists are sometimes vulnerable to "supermarket consultations" in any case, and if a neighbor-client-friend were to become hard to encounter in the grocery store because of the difficulty in setting limits on such informal consultations, this would constrict the therapist's life.

Guidelines.   Once the more obvious dual relationships to pose clear problems in maintaining objectivity and professional distance - such as those with family members, close friends, and coworkers and subordinates - have been eliminated from consideration, the therapist should ask himself or herself the following questions before accepting as a client an acquaintance, a friend of a friend, or someone whose status raises the potential for a social dual relationship:

1. Will the dual relationship inhibit in any way the client's ability to make autonomous decisions? Can you anticipate ways in which the client will feel that he or she cannot disagree with you because of outside demands of any sort?
2. Will the dual relationship restrict your response alternatives? Can you act the same way and say the same things that you would with any other client?
3. Where do your motivations fit in? Are you likely to find yourself playing to an imagined audience rather than doing what is clinically right? Will you be more tempted to be a hero to look good to your friends? Can you resist this temptation?

Because the temptation to accept a client in this type of context may be strong, it is important that the clinician honestly grapple with these considerations. Inherent in such deliberations is a tendency to rationalize, which should be acknowledged and examined as well.

FRIENDSHIPS WITH CLIENTS

Given the intimate nature of the therapeutic relationship and the amount of time a therapist spends with clients, it is not difficult to understand the temptation to develop friendships with clients and to want to socialize with them. Although such a temptation is natural, in general, we believe that such friendships should be avoided. A therapist-client relationship is based on trust, intimacy, and self-disclosure. Typically, the information flow goes one way. That is, the client shares much more personal information than does the therapist. The therapist, in turn, assumes an expert role - as one who is capable of handling such information sensitively and of being able to help the client.

This type of role definition has several consequences. Because of the time-limited and unique nature of the therapeutic relationship, a client is likely to self-disclose more than he or she would in a social relationship. An ongoing social relationship with a therapist, or the potential of one, may limit the client's perceived options in terms of how much to disclose. Further, it is unlikely that the therapist could act freely as a therapist and as a friend simultaneously; one relationship or the other would have to suffer. Perhaps the therapeutic relationship would break down in favor of a more symmetrical friendship, or the asymmetry of the therapeutic relationship would characterize the friendship; or there may be elements of both.

Although these contentions may be sensible to consider during the process of therapy, one may assert that once therapy is terminated, there should be nothing to stand in the way of a social relationship. In contrast, we believe that the process of therapy in most cases prevents a truly symmetrical social relationship from ever being able to develop. The fact that the friendship had its genesis in a therapeutic relationship will make it impossible to know what the nature of the friendship would have been otherwise, and the freedom of action of both participants is likely to be limited in very subtle ways. There is a question as to whether the ex-client could ever see the therapist in an objective light. It appears likely instead that there would always be some degree of distortion in the ex-client's view of the therapist. Further, if a social relationship is allowed to follow therapy, this is likely to preclude the possibility of that person's ever coming back into therapy with that therapist.

For the preceding reasons, the wise clinician should take appropriate steps to prevent the development of a friendship with a client, either during therapy or afterwards. This does not necessarily mean a rigid avoidance of social contact, but rather an expanded awareness of the potential for trouble.

GIFTS FROM CLIENTS

There are a number of reasons that a client may give a therapist a gift (Drew, Stoeckle, & Billings, 1983). At times, gift giving can be an honest and sincere expression of appreciation for the help a therapist has provided. At other times, however, a gift may be given for more functional reasons, for example, as a bid for a more social relationship with the therapist or as a means of asking the therapist to "go easy" on the client. There are also times when a gift is given as an out-and-out bribe - for instance, to motivate the therapist to write a helpful disability or workers' compensation evaluation.

It is not unethical in all situations to accept a gift from a client. In fact, it would be inappropriate and countertherapeutic to refuse a gift in some situations. On the other hand, accepting a gift would be clearly unethical in other situations. A number of factors should be considered in deciding whether or not to accept a gift from a client:

1. What are the client's apparent motives for giving the gift? Does there seem to be any ulterior motive, either overt or covert, that applies? For instance, does the client need something from the therapist, such as a positive letter to a court, or does the client want to control the type of feedback he or she hears from the therapist?
2. Will the gift have an effect on treatment? Although it is tempting to contend that the gift will have no impact on what the clinician says or does, a more honest analysis of feelings may reveal otherwise.
3. What is the value of the gift? It is easier to justify accepting a gift of little financial value than one of greater worth. Not only is the absolute cost of the gift relevant,

but also the proportion of the client's income that the gift represents. A gift worth $25 may represent a significant proportion of the income of a single mother living on welfare, but perhaps only a token when given by a wealthy person.

4. What about the temporal context? A gift given during the holiday season or at the end of therapy may have a different meaning from one given at some random time, or one accompanied by a statement such as "I just saw this and it reminded me of you."

At times, a therapist may feel uncomfortable about accepting a gift but may not know how to refuse it or give it back without hurting the client or being countertherapeutic. Following are some suggestions on how to refuse a gift without being unduly rejecting or causing undue embarrassment to the client.

1. Express a positive, caring sentiment to the client, such as, "I'm flattered by this, and pleased that you would feel so positive about your counseling experience, but I can't accept your generosity." ("Why not?" will be the response.)

2. Take responsibility for not being able to accept the gift, such as, "I know that you are giving me this in a positive, generous spirit, and I appreciate that, but in my experience therapy will go better if gifts aren't involved in our work."

3. Be deliberate and sensitive about how you clinically process the gift giving. Whereas you may want to tuck it away and bring it up thematically later, a client is likely to feel hurt and rejected if your first response is, "This seems to be one more way in which you try to buy acceptance."

4. Suggest an alternative that allows the client to express gratitude without the therapist benefiting directly, for example, "Since I can't accept this piano, if you sincerely want to express your gratitude about the help you've gotten, you may want to donate it to the Children's Hospital."

5. Be relaxed. If the clinician conveys a sense of discomfort
    and uncertainty about how to handle the gift, the client is
    likely to feel uncertain and uncomfortable as well. If you
    sense that a client may be planning to give you a gift, plan
    how you will respond, even to the point of rehearsing
    what you will say.

SEXUAL RELATIONSHIPS

In terms of sexual relationships with clients, ethical standards
are clear: Sex with a current client is unethical. This is specifically prohibited by the ethical standards of psychologists, psychiatrists, social workers, and marriage and family counselors. Further, sex does not merely mean sexual intercourse. Rather, it is
any form of intimate physical contact, such as kissing or fondling
(Bouhoutsos et al., 1983).

When evaluated in terms of the problems with dual relationships listed previously, it is apparent that sex is such a powerful
motivating factor that it is impossible to be objective about it. A
client's right to make autonomous decisions would certainly be
limited by a therapist who made a sexual advance. The therapist's
elevated power position, combined with the fact that the client
expects the therapist to act in a fiduciary capacity, make it virtually impossible for a client to make an autonomous decision regarding sexual involvement. Sonne and Pope (1991) found that
clients who have engaged in sex with their therapists respond in
ways similar to incest victims, feeling a sense of betrayal of trust,
role confusion, guilt, and so on.

In addition to the fact that clients have clearly diminished
capacities to make autonomous decisions in matters of sexual
relationships with therapists, it is also virtually impossible for a
therapist to be objective about sex with clients. Although a clinician might rationalize that a sexual involvement was somehow
therapeutic for the client, he or she could not separate the therapeutic aspects of the act from other aspects springing from his or
her personal motivations. The process of distinguishing clinical
from personal issues is always a concern in therapy, and the con-

sequences of being wrong are especially severe when sexual matters are concerned.

An area of greater confusion and disagreement relates to sex with former clients. Whereas it is generally agreed that sexual contact with a current client represents an unethical dual relationship, the issue becomes more complex after termination. One line of reasoning would say that a prohibition against sex with a former client restricts the client's autonomy. That is, to prohibit an individual from having sexual contact with his or her former therapist implies that, by the mere fact of having been a client, that individual has sacrificed his or her right to make autonomous decisions. Proponents of such a view would say that prohibition of sexual contact with a former client does not speak very highly of our attitudes toward our clients' decision-making ability or our view of the effectiveness of therapy.

According to another line of reasoning, "Once a client, always a client." Such a position holds that the same factors that make sex with a current client unethical would also apply to a former client. That is, just because a client has terminated, there is no proof that he or she will immediately develop an objective and symmetrical view of the therapist, nor does it seem likely that the therapist would immediately become completely objective in his or her view of the client. In addition, unpublished studies cited by the Ethics Committee of the American Psychological Association (1988) suggest that not only do clients create an internalized "image" of their therapist but also that the vividness and use of this image after termination is correlated with measures of improvement. The same source cites research to show that even in successfully terminated therapies, there tends to be a "gradual working through of the unresolved transference issues with passage of time following the treatment" and that the 5- to 10-year period following therapy would seem to be a critical time in the posttherapeutic development.

The various professional associations and state licensing boards have struggled and continue to struggle with the issue of sex with former clients (Sell, Gottlieb, & Schoenfield, 1986). Some ethical codes have been revised to accommodate the current emphasis on this issue. The current psychiatric version of the *Principles of*

Medical Ethics (American Psychiatric Association, 1993) has added the following statement, "Sexual activity with a current or former patient is unethical" (§2.1).

The *Ethical Principles of Psychologists and Code of Conduct* (American Psychological Association, 1992) has added a new section on sexual intimacies with former therapy patients. It states, "psychologists do not engage in sexual intimacies with former therapy patients and clients even after a two-year interval except in the most unusual circumstances" (§4.07b). Psychologists who do engage in sexual intimacies after the 2-year period following termination bear a special obligation to demonstrate that there has been no exploitation.

As noted earlier, the AAMFT *Code of Ethics* (1991) states, "Sexual intimacy with former clients for two years following the termination of therapy is prohibited" (§1.2).

We support an extremely conservative view regarding sex with former clients. Whereas a clinician could make a case that such involvement is ethically and clinically acceptable in a certain case, we believe that, in virtually all cases, the chances for exploitation or restriction of autonomy are extremely high because there are so many factors that could complicate the judgment of both individuals involved. We consider it wise, therefore, for the clinician to adopt the position of "Once a client, always a client."

GENERAL GUIDELINES

Previously, we offered suggestions regarding some of the issues a clinician should consider before proceeding in various contexts that have the potential for dual relationships. Of course, it would be difficult to address every potential dual relationship. Below are some general considerations for avoiding problematic dual relationships.

1. Any type of sexual contact with clients is unethical, as is conducting a professional relationship with a close friend, family member, coworker, or other person in a similarly intimate role.

2. For ethical (and legal) reasons, the clinician would be wise to adopt the position that sexual intimacies with a former client should always be avoided.

3. Ethical therapists are sensitive to their impact on clients. What may seem to be an innocuous comment may have significant impact on a client because of the regard in which the therapist is held.

4. Make the fulfillment of personal needs subordinate to the needs of the client. It is understandable that therapists derive emotional satisfaction of various sorts from their interactions with their clients. For the most part, such needs as being helpful and effective are appropriate. Therapists' other needs, such as needs for affection, emotional support, control, sexual gratification, or status should not be a part of the therapeutic context. Overtly or covertly using clients to meet such needs is counter-therapeutic. In this regard, it is highly advisable for therapists to be sure that they have extra-therapeutic options for meeting their emotional and physical needs. A therapist whose social outlets are too limited is very likely to rely too heavily on his or her clients for emotional fulfillment. The likelihood of making ill-advised clinical decisions or making inappropriate demands on a client is thus significantly increased.

   There are a few "early warning" signs that a therapist might be attempting to meet inappropriate needs with a client. These include an inordinate level of self-disclosure, excessive in spite of one's "better judgment"; the eager anticipation of particular clients' sessions; wishes to prolong sessions or the course of treatment despite having accomplished the major goals of therapy; and wishes (or actions) to please, impress, or punish the client.

5. When in doubt, consult trusted associates. Dual relationships are among the ethical issues about which it is most difficult to be objective, so therapists should not hesitate to seek consultation and should be receptive to the feedback received.

Chapter 7

Paternalism:
Exercising Power
Judiciously and
Promoting Client Autonomy

Consider the case of a private practitioner who sees an elderly male client for an initial interview. The client states that he has been communicating telepathically with Linda Ronstadt and that, through the radio, she has told him to give his life savings to charity. Should the therapist take steps to have a conservator appointed, that is, to have this man declared incompetent to manage his own funds? Should the therapist notify the client's family, regardless of his stated preferences? Should the therapist simply discuss the pros and cons of the intended action?

Consider an additional case: An adult client tells the therapist that she has been hoarding her antidepressant medication because she is thinking of killing herself. She mentions that she is sharing this information only because she knows the rules of confidentiality. Should the therapist take steps toward emergency commitment?

The preceding cases illustrate a conflict, commonly experienced in clinical practice, between the principle of autonomy and the principle of beneficence. As described by many writers in both mental health and philosophy (e.g., Faden & Beauchamp, 1986; Levine & Lyon-Levine, 1984), the principle of autonomy underscores human beings' right to determine their own goals, because it treats individual freedom as a crucial component of human affairs. The implication of this in clinical work is that therapist and client enter into a contractual relationship as two equals.   The principle of autonomy implies that the client is treated as an independent agent whose own goals are paramount, and that the therapist should help the client define and achieve those goals.   In contrast, the principle of beneficence underscores the promotion of human welfare as an ultimate good.   Acting in accord with this principle means that persons can sometimes be forced to do what is in their best interests.   The implication of this principle in clinical practice is that practitioners' perceptions of the best interests of the client may take precedence over clients' wishes.   This is typically referred to as paternalistic intervention.   The reasoning behind this is that the practitioner has the professional knowledge and judgment to know what is best for the client regardless of the client's wishes.

A clinician can take a number of actions that would be considered paternalistic.   Hospitalizing a mentally ill or suicidal client against his or her will, revealing confidential information to a family member to protect a client, and withholding diagnostic or treatment information from a client would all be considered paternalistic acts if carried out *because* the therapist believed that this was in the client's best interests, *and* the client would have preferred another course of action.   In all these cases, the practitioner has made a decision in what he or she thinks is the client's best interests, in spite of the client's preferences to the contrary.

This chapter deals with various aspects of paternalism.   The first section discusses some of the general ethical issues relevant to the beneficence-autonomy dimension.   Several clinical situations in which the question of paternalism is especially relevant are then described.   Finally, some guidelines are presented to help the clinician structure his or her decision making regarding paternalism.

ETHICAL ISSUES
RELATED TO PATERNALISM

The codes of ethics of the various mental health disciplines make general reference to situations in which a clinician can appropriately act paternalistically.   Thus, they imply that there may be contexts in which acting paternalistically is justified ethically. On the other hand, a number of explicit statements in the codes of ethics urge the practitioner to be diligent in safeguarding various client rights, such as in obtaining informed consent, the right of control over the confidentiality of communication, and so on. The *Code of Ethics* of the National Association of Social Workers (1993) states specifically that "The social worker should make every effort to foster maximum self-determination on the part of clients" (§II.G.).

These standards are all based on a respect for clients as individuals who can make their own decisions and act in their own best interests. The clear implication of these standards is that the clients' right to autonomy is the overriding principle. Although the practitioner may be ethical in acting paternalistically, the situations in which he or she does so must be well justified.

The following sections discuss paternalism in clinical settings and situations in which we believe the therapist may appropriately act to restrict the client's autonomy in some way. Such situations include those in which the client must be protected, in which society must be protected from the client, and in which there may be justification for withholding diagnostic or treatment information from the client.

PROTECTION OF THE CLIENT

INCOMPETENCE OR DISABILITY

As mentioned previously, the client should be afforded the maximum autonomy possible. However, at times, the client may display some form of disability that indicates that the practitioner's judgment should override the client's. There is little ethical ambiguity in the more obvious cases of clients who are so severely impaired because of thought disorder, mood disorder, or organic brain syndrome that they would be in immediate danger of self-harm. In such cases, the clinician should intervene to hospitalize the client, notify family members, or take some other action to protect the client's well-being, regardless of the patient's preferences. However, the question remains: At what level of disability is the practitioner justified in limiting the client's decision-making options? In the preceding vignette concerning the man who believed he was commanded by Linda Ronstadt to give his money to charity, would the clinician be justified in notifying a family member, attempting to have the client declared incompetent, or taking some other step to limit the client's freedom?

As described earlier, in dealing with these questions it is assumed that the client's right of autonomy will prevail unless the practitioner can justify breaching this right. In making a decision to take a paternalistic step, a number of questions should be considered. The reader may find it useful to see if the following guidelines provide direction in how to deal with the client in the vignette just mentioned.

1. *What is the disabling condition that you feel justifies paternalism?* The practitioner should be able to document the reasons the client cannot make his or her own decision. It is not enough to state that the client has "poor judgment." There should be some identifiable condition, such as schizophrenia or organic brain syndrome, that limits the client's decision-making ability.

2. *Are there legal guidelines?* The practitioner needs to be aware of prevailing laws and court decisions, particularly statutes regarding the conditions under which involuntary commitment is mandated. Further, the practitioner should know, or be able to find, the statutory definition of competence. Competence to make contracts, competence to stand trial, and competence to administer one's own financial affairs are, for example, common domains in which statutory limitations exist. These limitations vary by state, and can be located by reviewing state law or consulting a knowledgeable attorney.

3. *What negative effects would occur if you did not take paternalistic action?* If the client is likely only to make an unwise decision, paternalism becomes harder to justify. However, if failure to act were likely to result in death or serious harm, then paternalistic action would become more justifiable.

4. *Is there a less controlling step?* It may be possible to deal with the issue in a way that safeguards the client's autonomy, possibly in a clinically beneficial manner. For instance, if there is concern about whether the client can care for himself or herself, rather than immediately beginning commitment proceedings, it may be desirable to discuss available options with the client and come up with a mutually satisfactory solution. In the case of the elderly client discussed previously, less controlling actions might include the following: The therapist may ask the client for permission to include the family in sessions to discuss the proper handling of his finances, or the therapist could vigorously encourage the client to wait until a thorough discussion had taken place before acting.

SUICIDE

Good clinical practice suggests that the clinician pay attention to signs that predict suicide and act accordingly; the clinician could be guilty of malpractice if he or she overlooks such signs (R. L. Schwitzgebel & R. K. Schwitzgebel, 1980; Swenson, 1986). However, consider the case in which a client does not have a disabling mental condition that would inhibit his or her decision-making ability, seems rational and objective, yet shows evidence of suicidal intent. Does the practitioner have an obligation to try to stop such a client from committing suicide in such a situation?

Philosophically and ethically speaking, a case could be made that under appropriate circumstances, the right to commit suicide is part of the individual's right to autonomy. A number of writers (e.g., Szasz, 1986) have made such a point. On the other hand, suicide is an irrevocable step, driven by complex motivation. This makes it difficult to determine whether an individual is actually making a free, autonomous decision to commit suicide.

It is also difficult to conceive of very many clinicians who, even if they philosophically believed that suicide was an individual's right, could allow a client to leave their office intending suicide. Such behavior would likely be inconsistent with most clinicians' personal ethical frameworks. Typically, there is something clinically meaningful about a patient's disclosure of suicidal intentions, and the clinician must balance his or her ethical and legal obligations with a clinical awareness. The clinical significance of a client telling a therapist (who is obviously committed to preserving life) of his or her desire to end life must be carefully considered. Indeed, as Hoffman (1979) has provocatively argued, it may be clinically inappropriate to respond to a patient's disclosure of suicidal intentions with a paternalistic intervention such as beginning commitment proceedings.

These issues are obviously very complex. In addition to the ethical decision about "allowing" a client to commit suicide (or not taking steps to prevent it), there is a legal aspect to the issue. Ethical codes and legal case precedent make it clear that therapists are not only permitted to act paternalistically in the interests of preserving their clients' lives, but they could be considered professionally negligent if they fail to take any steps at all (Berman & Cohen-Sandler, 1983; Cohen & Mariano, 1982). If, in the clinician's best professional judgment, the issue can be dealt with clinically and nonpaternalistically without undue risk to the patient's life, then he or she is usually justified in proceeding clinically. However, if the clinician believes that the patient represents a serious suicide risk, then some appropriate action must be taken or the clinician will be acting negligently.

PROTECTION OF OTHERS

At times a practitioner's obligations to clients may be secondary to his or her societal obligations. However, it is not technically paternalism when a practitioner intervenes to keep a client from hurting someone else; defining an intervention as paternalistic implies that the practitioner is acting in the best interests of the client, not protecting others. Still, it requires only a small stretch of the concept to argue that, in fact, the therapist does help the patient by removing some of his or her freedom to act violently toward others. In addition, of course, the therapist acts to protect third parties who may be potential victims. Some have argued that the concept should not be stretched this far - in fact, society should not expect therapists to do detective work in addition to psychological healing (e.g., Bersoff, 1976). Nonetheless, because the demands made on practitioners in such cases are similar to those placed on them when a paternalistic action is being considered, a discussion of protection of others is appropriate here.

Much has been written about clinicians' legal obligations to protect others from the actions of a client (e.g., Cohen & Mariano, 1982; Kaufman, 1991; Knapp & VandeCreek, 1982). Here, we will present a brief summary of relevant legal issues, followed by a discussion of some of the important ethical considerations.

VIOLENCE

The *Tarasoff* decision (*Tarasoff v. Board of Regents of University of California*, 1976) established the obligation of the therapist to protect potential victims of their clients' violence. Although this decision has been interpreted as developing a "duty to warn," such breaching of confidentiality is only one of the options available to the practitioner as part of the broader "duty to protect." Other alternatives include hospitalizing the client, modifying the environment so that danger is reduced (such as requiring the client to get rid of lethal weapons), or bringing the potential victim into therapy to resolve problem issues (Knapp & VandeCreek, 1982).

In most cases, for the "duty to protect" to apply, the practitioner must know (or should have known based on prevailing standards of practice) that a client presents an immediate danger to an identifiable person. If there is a high likelihood of violence but no identifiable victim, then the practitioner's options are limited primarily to hospitalization. Several "negligent release" cases have been brought on the grounds that persons dangerous in general should be confined and treated to protect the community at large (Cohen & Mariano, 1982). For the most part, however, court decisions have found therapists negligent more for failure to assess their patients' past histories of violent or dangerous behavior than for their inability to predict dangerousness or violent behavior in the future (Applebaum, 1985). On the other hand, courts have also decided that failure to take action in response to what should have been evidence of violent tendencies is negligent or incompetent (e.g., *Peck v. The Counseling Service of Addison County*, 1985; *Petersen v. State*, 1983).

It is difficult to arrive at a single prevailing standard emerging from the various cases that have followed *Tarasoff.* Outcomes are often contradictory or inconsistent. Felthous (1989) has made the point that the states must enact statutes clearly delineating therapists' responsibilities vis-à-vis dangerous clients. At least 16 states have enacted statutes that have limited the therapist's *Tarasoff* obligations in various ways (Kaufman, 1991).

In summarizing state statutes and case law, it is safe to say that clinicians have an obligation to be aware of any potential for violence on the part of their clients, also considering any past incidents of violence, and to take justifiable steps that are in the best interests of both clients and potential victims. If the client is not committable by prevailing statutes, then the best strategy available to the practitioner may be to maintain the therapeutic relationship and attempt to work on the issues in that context.

PHYSICAL AND SEXUAL ABUSE

All 50 states have statutes mandating reporting of suspected physical or sexual abuse of a minor (Butz, 1985). If the survey of psychologists conducted by Haas, Malouf, and Mayerson (1986) is representative of other mental health professions, the practitioners seem well aware of this requirement. Given the number of times that mandatory reporting questions arise, it is important that clinicians know the prevailing statutes in their jurisdictions. It is particularly important that the clinician know (or be able to find) the pertinent definitions of such terms as physical and sexual abuse, incest, and molestation, because knowledge of these definitions is critical in helping a practitioner make a decision as to appropriate action in a given situation.

ETHICAL CONSIDERATIONS
IN PROTECTING OTHERS

Although it appears that practitioners commonly know their legal obligations in the circumstances described previously, obeying the law does not necessarily guarantee that the clinician will be acting ethically. A number of ethical concerns should be addressed by the clinician in the process of defining appropriate actions. The first of these relates to breaching confidentiality. Given prevailing legal requirements and precedents, it may seem that the practitioner is more likely to avoid malpractice suits by routinely reporting any potential violence or any suspected physical or sexual abuse, especially because statutes typically grant immunity from liability to anyone who reports suspected abuse in good faith. Unfortunately, this strategy has ethical shortcomings. Specifically, given our tendency to overpredict violence, a reporting policy that is too liberal may violate the rights of confidentiality of many individuals who are likely to harm no one and waste the resources of child protection agencies. In fact, the reporting process may damage reputations and relationships. Such concerns must be counterbalanced against the clinician's legal and ethical obligations to protect innocent parties.

Consequently, we recommend that practitioners consider the ethical, as well as the legal, ramifications of their decisions and assiduously avoid a "knee-jerk" reporting strategy. Practitioners should report what they are required to report to protect others, and no more. Consultation with other professionals would obviously prove valuable in questionable situations.

Another significant ethical consideration relates to a major theme in this chapter, namely, the importance of safeguarding client autonomy. Even when a decision is made to breach confidentiality or override client desires in another way, there may be means of increasing the client's sense of self-direction. For instance, many clinicians give clients the option of reporting physical or sexual abuse themselves. Likewise, in cases of potential violence, clients should, when appropriate, participate in the process of deciding how to assure the safety of the threatened individual. It has even been noted (Beck, 1982) that this involvement may contribute to the patient's remaining in treatment versus dropping out. Only when circumstances demand should decisions be made without the client's knowledge and participation. For example, if a particular client is so paranoid and out of control that his or her motivation and ability to improve the situation cannot be trusted, the clinician may decide to exclude him or her from the process of protecting others, even if his or her autonomy is restricted in the process.

WITHHOLDING DIAGNOSTIC OR
TREATMENT INFORMATION

Possibly the most commonly encountered aspect of paternalism relates to withholding information regarding a client's diagnosis or treatment plan. If this information is not made available, the client's autonomy is reduced. He or she lacks the information required to make such decisions as whether or not to receive treatment, what form of treatment to participate in, and so on. Obviously, this issue overlaps that of informed consent, and much of what is presented in Chapter 5 is relevant here.

Dawson (1981) lists a number of reasons that therapists withhold or distort information. Among these are the client's perceived inability to understand relevant information because of its technical nature, the fact that diagnostic and treatment information is always uncertain in psychotherapy, clients' lack of desire to know, incapacity of the client to be informed, resistance of the therapist, and nonmaleficence (i.e., the therapist's wish to avoid harming the client). In reviewing the justifications for each of these reasons, Dawson concludes that there is typically very little justification for withholding "autonomy-relevant" information or for deceiving clients. Only two situations justify withholding information: when the client's disability prevents him or her from being able to understand or make decisions based on relevant information, or when the practitioner determines that the knowledge would be harmful to the client.

The implication for practice is that clients should be given access to all relevant information unless there is a good reason for it to be withheld. If a client has some incapacity that clearly limits his or her ability to understand or make appropriate decisions, then the clinician has the option, and often the obligation, to withhold information.

With regard to nonmaleficence, it is important that practitioners be very deliberate in defining situations in which full disclosure of information would be countertherapeutic or harmful to the client in some other way. As Dawson mentions, a number of factors can produce positive outcomes in therapy, such as the placebo effect, an optimistic attitude on the part of the therapist, and the therapist's ability to stimulate confidence and trust. To the extent that withholding certain information enhances these factors, doing so may be ethically justifiable. However, at the same time, the clinician should be constantly aware of the client's right to make autonomous decisions and include this factor in his or her decision making as well.

Further, it is critical that the clinician not confuse nonmaleficence and convenience. That is, the decision to withhold relevant treatment information should be based on avoiding harm to the client rather than on what is easiest for the therapist. Generally, decisions to withhold information tend to result from therapists' concerns that clients will become upset or even leave treatment as a result. Consider, for example, a case in which the therapist believes that treatment will be very lengthy and the client asks "How long will we need to meet?" A therapist who avoids this question may possibly believe that it would be disturbing to a client to realize that he or she is a "long-term case." Perhaps the therapist believes that there is no effective way to truthfully answer the question. However, the likely motivation in such cases may well be the desire not to commit oneself or get "locked in" to a specific treatment duration. In the former case, paternalistic action is justified on the basis of client welfare. That is, the potentially resistant client may be better able to hear the information at a later time. In the latter case, it is possible that self-interest, rather than paternalism, is the real issue.

Alternatively, consider the case of a therapist who is asked, "Have you ever seen anyone like me before?" and who indeed has not. If the situation is not similar to that discussed in Chapter 3, in which referral or supervision is indicated, then the question of paternalism versus nonmaleficence arises. Telling the client that one is new to his or her problem may undermine faith in treatment (unless it is done in such a way that the client becomes a "team member" and collaborates on treatment).

CONCLUSION AND
RECOMMENDATIONS

Because paternalism can subtly intrude on clinical practice, practitioners should periodically question themselves (or have colleagues question them) about ways in which the same clinical end could be achieved without sacrificing client autonomy. Perhaps because of a lower frustration tolerance, medicalization of clinical practice, or gradual loss of humility, practitioners can find it easier to "do for" the client instead of facilitating the client's "doing for" himself or herself. We are not advocating abandonment of one's responsibility to clients. Rather, we suggest that periodic attention to this issue is not only of ethical importance, but can lend an elegance and authority to therapy that is not easily achieved any other way.

Chapter 8

Loyalty Conflicts:
Balancing Professional
and Organizational Demands

Loyalty conflicts may be defined as situations in which a practitioner bears a professional obligation to one or more parties, and these obligations are contradictory in some way. The practitioner is thus in a position of having to establish priorities for professional loyalties and responsibilities. Such conflicts can emerge in both subtle and overt ways. Unfortunately, the ethical standards of the various mental health disciplines offer little specific guidance in terms of practical decision making regarding loyalty conflicts. Beyond fairly general statements such as "The social worker's primary responsibility is to clients" (NASW, 1993, §II.F.), practitioners are largely left to their own devices.

This chapter is devoted to the question of loyalty conflicts in professional practice. Four general categories of loyalty conflicts are highlighted, along with some of the specific considerations of each. The types of loyalty conflicts to be discussed include conflicts based on difficulty defining the client, conflicts between loyalty to the client and loyalty to one's organization, conflicts between loyalty to the client and appropriate standards of professional practice, and conflicts between loyalty to the client and the law.

LOYALTY CONFLICTS BASED ON
DIFFICULTY IN DEFINING THE CLIENT

In the simplest case, the client is both the focus of service (e.g., evaluation, therapy) and the source of payment. If these are two different individuals or entities, then the issues become more problematic. Questions arise concerning such issues as ownership of information, rights of confidentiality, where the practitioner's responsibilities lie when the parties conflict, and so on. This problem has been most thoroughly explored with regard to the dilemmas psychologists face when being hired to provide psychological services in the criminal-justice system (see Monahan, 1980).

However, similar problems exist for other professionals and in other aspects of clinical practice. Consider the following example. An attorney contacts a psychotherapist because she has a female client (sole custodian of the children) whose ex-husband is suing for visitation rights. The woman has reason to believe that her ex-husband is emotionally unstable, and her attorney requests that the clinician evaluate the ex-husband and bill the ex-wife. Could information be released about the ex-husband without a signed release of information from him? Would he even have access to the results of his own evaluation? Similar questions arise when a business hires a practitioner to provide services to its employees, and even when a parent hires a practitioner to provide services to a minor child. If something revealed by the person receiving services is relevant to the party paying the bill, where do the practitioner's loyalties lie? Another example of such potential conflict is the case of a worker who reveals to her therapist, who is paid by the worker's employer, that she is embezzling funds.

In our reading of current ethical standards and available literature, we find little that a practitioner can fall back on to help make decisions in these situations. In the ethical standards of the various mental health professions, the most directly pertinent statement is found in the *Ethical Principles of Psychologists and Code of Conduct* (American Psychological Association, 1992), in which Section 1.21 states:

(a) When a psychologist agrees to provide services to a person or entity at the request of a third party, the psychologist clarifies to the extent feasible, at the outset of the service, the nature of the relationship with each party. This clarification includes the role of the psychologist (such as therapist, organizational consultant, diagnostician, or expert witness), the probable uses of the services provided or the information obtained, and the fact that there may be limits to confidentiality.

(b) If there is a foreseeable risk of the psychologist's being called upon to perform conflicting roles because of the involvement of a third party, the psychologist clarifies the nature and direction of his or her responsibilities, keeps all parties appropriately informed as matters develop, and resolves the situation in accordance with the Ethics Code.

This would suggest that prevention is the best remedy for conflict. That is, practitioners should anticipate the interests and expectations that all parties might have in a particular situation and act in ways that would minimize misunderstanding and failed expectations. What this means specifically varies from situation to situation, but in general, the practitioner should assess each party's stake in the action, define the conditions under which the confidentiality of the recipient of services would be breached, negotiate and obtain agreement on the nature and extent of information sharing, and so on. As part of this process, the practitioner may seek consultation regarding the legal aspects of the case. There may be legal constraints within which the practitioner must act and which must be embodied in whatever arrangement is negotiated.

A guiding principle in such negotiations is respect for the privacy of an individual and for the confidentiality of the information that may be shared. This guideline suggests that information should be revealed only to the extent necessary to accomplish the purpose at hand. For example, in a case in which one partner is paying for the evaluation of another, there is no need to share personal information that does not pertain to the question at hand;

to share such information would represent an unnecessary violation of an individual's right to privacy.

To summarize, whereas ethical guidelines contain no specific information about how to resolve dilemmas created by multiple clients with different demands, it is suggested that the practitioner be open about the issues involved, try to anticipate the needs and demands of each party, and negotiate acceptable arrangements in advance. The ideal result of such negotiations would be a plan that reflects the needs of each party, relevant legal guidelines, and, to the extent possible, respect for privacy and confidentiality. A less-than-ideal outcome of such negotiations may bring the practitioner to the conclusion that the parties' different needs cannot be reconciled. In such cases it is better to withdraw as a possible service provider (or to include additional providers) than to accept an impossible contract in the hopes that positions will change.

LOYALTY TO THE CLIENT VERSUS
LOYALTY TO ONE'S ORGANIZATION

Situations may arise in which the purported needs of the client conflict with the needs of the practitioner's employing agency or organization. A number of such situations may occur, such as being requested by an agency director to refer a client to a therapist one does not trust, or being asked to terminate a client who has not paid a bill.

When faced with such questions, what are practitioners' options? Are they ethically bound to honor the client's needs, even if they conflict with the needs of the organization, or can clinicians be ethical and still support such organizational needs, even to the detriment of a client? Again, ethical guidelines make few specific statements relevant to this question. The *Ethical Principles of Psychologists and Code of Conduct* (American Psychological Association, 1992) makes this statement:

> If the demands of an organization with which psychologists are affiliated conflict with this Ethics Code, psychologists clarify the nature of the conflict, make known their commitment to the Ethics Code, and to the extent feasible,

seek to resolve the conflict in a way that permits the fullest adherence to the Ethics Code. (§8.03)

Although this statement is vague, it clearly does not state the expectation that psychologists obey the ethical principles above all else. In other words, psychologists do not have the obligation to commit professional suicide to uphold the code of ethics. The principle does mandate, however, that psychologists make sure that the issues are clear to concerned individuals, including the fact that there is an ethical concern, and that they attempt to comply with the ethical principles as closely as feasible (leaving it up to the psychologist to define "feasible").

By extension, and in the absence of relevant sections of other ethical codes, these concepts can be applied by other practitioners. Much is left to the discretion of the practitioner when the needs of the organization seem to be opposed to those of the client. Following are descriptions of two types of situations in which the practitioner is confronted with such conflicting loyalties.

LOYALTY CONFLICTS RELATING TO CLIENT CONFIDENTIALITY

Consider the situation in which a client tells her therapist at a mental health center that she has not been taking the medication prescribed by the staff psychiatrist. Or consider a situation in which a patient at an agency that sets fees on a sliding scale tells the therapist that he makes more money than he initially reported. If proper procedures for providing information necessary to obtain informed consent have been followed (see Chapter 5), then the client has been led to believe that the therapist will maintain complete confidentiality (with the exception of legal requirements such as mandatory reporting). This places the clinician in an ethical conflict regarding whether to reveal confidential information to other members of the organization without the expressed consent of the client. Although customary practice allows for some necessary sharing of information when appropriate, clients may, not unreasonably, expect to have their confidences respected.

In dealing with situations such as the ones discussed previously, the clinician does have certain options. The first, of course, would be to anticipate such problems and include specific statements related to them in a consent form signed by the client. Second, the situation can be handled as a clinical issue (e.g., dealing with it as the client's request for limits). Third, the clinician may strongly assert that he or she needs to share the confidential information with the appropriate individual(s) within the organization and try to elicit the patient's consent to do so. If such consent is not forthcoming, the practitioner may decide that effective therapy with the client is impossible under the circumstances (e.g., the client's unwillingness to allow coordination among clinical personnel, or personal feelings aroused by the client's deceptiveness). In such a case, termination or transfer may be justifiable.

CONFLICTS BASED ON DISAGREEMENTS WITH ONE'S ORGANIZATION

The issue discussed before puts loyalty conflicts in a context in which the practitioner supports the organization's policies. What are a clinician's alternatives if he or she feels that the organization, or a representative thereof, is wrong? For instance, the clinician might determine that a client needs long-term therapy while the agency allows only six sessions; or the client clearly needs psychotropic medications and the agency director has a firm antimedication stance. In polling psychologists about a specific instance of this dilemma, Haas et al. (1986) found that the vast majority of psychologists stated that they would refuse to support the organizational policy if they disagreed with it. However, what people say they would do and what they would actually do in such situations might be different.

It would obviously be ethically unsound for a clinician to support a policy that he or she believed was harmful to the client. Such an action would be contrary to the practitioner's obligation to promote the client's welfare. At the same time, openly disagreeing with the policy may be destructive to the unity of the organization, as well as possibly countertherapeutic for the client. Resolving such a dilemma would require that the clinician exercise a significant amount of diplomacy, working to change the organization's position while not being openly critical of it with the client. The clinician would be wise to spend time trying to understand and clarify both his or her own and the agency's positions, searching for areas of possible compromise. If no mutually satisfactory resolution can be found, then the clinician is forced to make a decision to either support or contradict the organization's position and to deal with the consequences of the decision. This would likely be a no-win situation, so expending considerable effort to arrive at a mutually acceptable resolution of the problem would clearly be worth the time. For example, in the preceding illustration, the clinician might see the client pro bono (at no cost) while advocating for an exception with the director. The alternative of simply discharging the client and immediately picking him or her up again for another six sessions probably would be considered deceptive or manipulative and not contribute to a reasonable resolution. In the second example, the clinician could obviously refer the case to a more appropriate agency, but this leaves the policy unchanged. Perhaps the therapist could initiate a discussion among the staff regarding the wisdom of such an antimedication policy. This might enhance the chances of the director changing his or her mind. This type of dilemma is likely to present itself in the managed care arena, as the dictates of the patient's insurance plan often restrict treatment options although they do not restrict the therapist's obligation to provide treatment. Geraty, Hendren, and Flaa (1992) describe the increasing influence on the practice of child and adolescent psychiatry, for example, detailing provider liability in a managed health care context (*Wickline v. State of California*), in which ultimate responsibility for the proper treatment of a patient was placed on the treating physician. The insurance company was absolved in a suit of negligence brought by the patient (cf. also, Applebaum, 1993; discussion in Chapter 11).

CONFLICTS BETWEEN LOYALTY TO THE CLIENT AND APPROPRIATE STANDARDS OF PROFESSIONAL PRACTICE

At times clinicians may feel caught between what they believe to be in the best interest of a client and appropriate standards of professional practice. For example, a clinician may be working with a recently divorced woman who is emotionally healthy but who has no vocational skills nor any money to educate herself. For her to qualify for publicly sponsored rehabilitation services, it is necessary to document an emotional disorder of some sort, and the client may ask the therapist to do so. What are the clinician's options and responsibilities in such situations?

To further illustrate, a divorcing client may ask the clinician to come to court and testify that the client is the more effective parent and should be granted custody. Assuming that he or she has not met the spouse and thus can make no comparison, what options are available to the clinician? To accede to the client's wish would violate an important standard of professional practice in that a practitioner cannot responsibly make comparative statements when he or she has only met one of the spouses.

These conflicts often arise because of conflicting demands for objectivity and advocacy. Whereas standards of professional practice promote objectivity - asserting that the clinician is expected to diagnose accurately, practice within the bounds of the available data, and so on, clinicians are frequently seen by their clients as being advocates. Clinicians themselves are often drawn to the client-advocate role. Implied in this role can be expectations that the clinician will compromise professional standards in the service of client needs.

There is certainly room for debate regarding when to compromise standards of professional practice; however, our contention is that these standards should be compromised very rarely, if ever. There are several reasons for a stringently conservative view regarding this. The first is purely ethical. For example, in the case first cited previously, lying is inherently unethical, even though arguments for "tempering the truth" can and have been made. The burden of proof is obviously on a practitioner who distorts the truth to show why such an action is justified.

The second reason a conservative view is preferred involves the credibility of the mental health professions. If individuals freely compromise their professional judgment, even for what seem to be good reasons, the overall effect is a reduction in the public's trust of mental health workers as objective professionals. Increased stringency in insurance company reimbursements and decreased influence of mental health professionals in court, among others, are likely outcomes.

Clinical considerations comprise the third justification for a conservative stance. Although in the short run it may seem appropriate to sacrifice one's standards on behalf of a client, the precedent may have an overall deleterious effect on the therapeutic relationship. The impact of knowing that one's therapist compromised his or her own standards, no matter what the reason, may ultimately prove countertherapeutic. For example, such actions may create the expectation that the clinician will solve all of the client's problems, thus removing the responsibility for problem solving from the client.

With the above in mind, what should a clinician do if confronted with a conflict between ethical standards and client needs? First, clinicians should honestly assess their motivations. Is this truly an ethical conflict or is there some other motivation, such as desiring to avoid alienating a client or funding source, securing reimbursement, taking the path of least resistance, wanting to be admired, or the like? Second, the clinician should explore alternatives. Are there other, more professionally honest, ways of dealing with the problem? Third, the clinician should consider the negative impacts of compromising standards - on the client, on the relationship, and on psychotherapeutic practice in general. Only if the motivation is truly ethical, there are no alternatives, and the benefits outweigh the costs should the clinician consider sacrificing professional standards.

In the case first cited previously, the clinician could help the client search for a different rehabilitation program. It should also be noted that telling the truth in this type of case preserves one's credibility with the agency. Alternatively, one could, without distorting the truth, describe the likely results of failure to obtain the rehabilitation service. In the second case (evaluation to determine custody), the most professionally honest course would be to report only what one knows and to suggest appropriate, unbiased evaluations.

CONFLICTS BETWEEN LOYALTY
TO THE CLIENT AND THE LAW

The practitioner may feel himself or herself in a bind when confronted by a conflict between the obligation to obey the law and duty to the client. Such binds may be created by cases of mandatory reporting, duty to warn, responding to subpoenas, and related issues (see Chapters 4 and 7). If the clinician believes that obeying the law may not be in the client's best interest, then a true dilemma is created.

In deciding how to resolve such dilemmas, the practitioner could choose the safest course, always obeying the law. As long as the law is clear, well-understood, and appropriately followed, such a course may be justifiable. However, it is incumbent on the practitioner not to play it so safe that confidentiality is breached through reporting clinical information or responding to subpoenas when such action is not justified. For instance, although it may assuage the practitioner's anxiety to report to the authorities or family members any hint of suicide or physical aggressiveness raised in therapy, this is inappropriate unless the practitioner believes that such behavior is likely. Various sources (e.g., Cohen & Mariano, 1982; DeKraii & Sales, 1984; Knapp & VandeCreek, 1982) describe the conditions under which confidentiality may be breached.

Other practitioners may believe that slavish obedience to the law is not ethical (that good client care may be compromised by "overconforming"). The clinician, for instance, may believe it inappropriate to report a case of sexual molestation, thinking that doing so would alienate the client and interrupt the therapeutic process. Such noncompliance is very risky for a number of reasons. First, when the law establishes the conditions for violating a client's right to confidentiality, it is usually done to protect the security of innocent individuals. If the clinician does not abide by legal requirements, he or she is, in effect, assuming responsibility for the well-being of potential victims; if something does happen, the clinician bears the moral (and legal) responsibility. Given the inaccuracy of predicting behavior and the tendency to believe a client's assertions that any inappropriate behavior will not be repeated, the risk of disobeying the law is significant.

Another risk in disobeying the law is that a clinical mistake will likely be made. The credibility and professionalism of a clinician who violates a legal requirement is likely to be compromised, and, unfortunately, many clients would capitalize on this compromised position in service of their own needs. Also, by agreeing to keep a secret, the clinician may effectively buffer the client from dealing with the consequences of his or her own behavior and thus allow avoidance of responsibility.

In deciding whether or not to obey legal requirements, the clinician would thus be wise to adopt a very stringent standard and to consider a number of aspects, only some of which are the same as in the preceding section. First, the practitioner should assess his or her motivations. Is the temptation to disregard the law truly based on the best interest of the client, or are there other motivations, such as a desire not to make the client angry, a desire to avoid legal hassles, and so on? Second, is it clear that disobedience to the law is obviously the best course clinically? Third, can the clinician be willing to accept any consequences that result if the legal disobedience is brought to light? Such a decision-making process may reduce the number of conflicts between the professional's personal standards and the perceived demands of the law.

ETHICAL ISSUES IN MANAGED CARE

As all mental health practitioners are aware, in recent years there has been a consistent trend away from traditional fee-for-service models of health care toward managed care systems such as health maintenance organization (HMOs), preferred provider organizations (PPOs), and the like. These systems regulate the use of health care with "gatekeepers" and review the care provided to individual patients. They reserve the right to deny payment for care they deem medically unnecessary or excessive (Applebaum, 1993). It is likely that the trend toward such systems will, if anything, accelerate.

In addition to the financial, legal, and clinical concerns raised by managed care, the clinician must deal with a number of ethical concerns. These concerns have been discussed in the literature to a certain extent in recent years (e.g., the special issue of *Professional Psychology: Research and Practice* on managed care by Lowman, 1991). This section will highlight some of the major ethical issues and will attempt to provide some recommendations for practitioners struggling with these problems.

A primary ethical concern in dealing with the managed mental health care system is whether or not clients are able to receive mental health care that is appropriate to their needs and that is of sufficient intensity and duration. The ethical conflict centering on the financial incentive for reducing care is difficult to resolve. What responsibilities does the clinician incur when an external body approves and directs a client's treatment and when that external body may have incentives for limiting the amount of treatment provided? First, the clinician has the responsibility to insure that he or she has sought approval for an appropriate level of care and to provide the necessary documentation. In other words, the therapist must play by the rules if he or she has already agreed to do so. Second, if the managed care organization refuses to approve treatment that the clinician believes is necessary, the clinician should pursue the case through all necessary appeal steps. This is not only an ethically appropriate stance, but it may be legally prudent as well. The *Wickline* case (*Wickline v. State of California*, 1986) is illustrative in this regard. The clinician (in this case not a therapist) was held liable for failing to protest the HMO's denial of treatment to a man who later died from the illness. Third, the clinician has the ethical and often legal obligation to continue services even though payment may be terminated. The therapeutic obligation supersedes the financial contract.

The decision to join particular managemental health care plans is one that practitioners will increasingly face. Haas and Cummings (1991) discuss the issues prospective providers should consider. They urge that prospective providers know exactly what the plan involves and what constraints will be imposed. Specific questions concern the following:

1. *Who takes the risks?* If the practitioner takes the financial risk for services exceeding what was predicted (as is the case in HMO arrangements), there may be a temptation to limit services inappropriately.
2. *How much does the plan intrude into the patient/provider relationship?* As opposed to traditional fee-for-service

arrangements, managed care systems involve more intrusion into the therapeutic relationship. At the minimum this typically involves a much greater intrusion into confidentiality than in traditional arrangements. Practitioners must be able to balance loyalty to their patients with responsibilities as "agents" of the mental health care carrier.

3. *What provisions exist for appealing adverse rulings?* The clinician should consider the plan's options for extending treatment beyond the typical length of service approved by the plan.

4. *Are there referral resources if patient needs exceed plan benefits?* Although there is an obligation in all the mental health professions to avoid abandonment, there are practical limitations in terms of how many low-fee or no-fee cases a practitioner can afford to carry. The ethical clinician must consider how to avoid abandoning patients without going bankrupt (Applebaum, 1993).

5. *Is the plan open to provider input?* If there is no mechanism for the practitioner to provide feedback to the plan managers, then it is hard to characterize his or her role as that of a professional independently or autonomously treating patients. The clinician can have no assurance that the plan managers are indeed interested in delivering quality care, although this can be hoped for.

6. *Does the plan clearly inform policyholders about the limits of their benefits?* This is an issue of informed consent, but it is one which the therapist would be well advised to raise with prospective clients before they enter a treatment relationship.

Managed care arrangements are not inherently unethical and, in fact, may reduce certain ethical concerns such as the tendency to provide excessive services because one is reimbursed for them. Nonetheless, managed care systems do raise ethical problems, and the clinician involved with such systems would be wise to anticipate and deal with them in advance.

Chapter 9

Relationships With
Professional Colleagues

No mental health professional practices in isolation. Whether it is consultation with colleagues to improve the treatment of a particularly complex case, discussing professional norms, or simply becoming aware of how colleagues handle particular issues, we all spend a considerable portion of our professional lives in dialogue with colleagues in our own and related mental health professions. It is also the case that professions are defined as self-regulating groups of practitioners. That is, a substantial portion of the responsibility for maintaining professional standards falls on the professionals themselves. This means that not only do we as mental health practitioners have an ethical obligation to monitor our own behavior and take steps to deal with conflicts or personal problems that interfere with our effectiveness, but we also have the responsibility to work with colleagues who appear to be practicing at a substandard level. Conversely, when we ourselves are not functioning effectively or are making ethical errors, colleagues are often the first to notice. Because of these issues, the codes of all the mental health professionals underscore the obligation of practitioners to confront, when appropriate, their colleagues whose behavior is raising questions.

The actions one can take with regard to a colleague, however, are limited. A colleague may choose to do nothing when faced with evidence of substandard professional behavior on another's part; in fact, this is probably the typical response. Another frequently chosen response is discussing the problem with *other* colleagues without directly contacting the individual about whom there are questions. Third, a colleague may report the behavior to a formal regulatory body, although often there are questions about whether such a drastic action is appropriate - either because the severity of the behavior does not warrant formal action or because there is insufficient evidence available to an ethics committee or similar body.

In many situations, the preferred option is to contact the colleague directly with one's questions or concerns. Although this is a desirable option, it is also extremely difficult to implement. Defensiveness or denial on the part of the questioned clinician, fears that one will be the subject of a counter-accusation (after all, who feels completely certain of the purity of his or her own practice?), wishes that someone else would do the job, hopes that one has simply been misinformed - all these factors are obstacles to direct contact with possibly erring colleagues. Gary Schoener, an early worker in this area, has noted that psychologists are notoriously poor at giving each other direct feedback about concerns they may have (personal communication, 1989). Unfortunately, this is likely to hold true for other mental health disciplines as well.

Questions surrounding the propriety of confronting colleagues about suspected unethical or substandard practices and questions about one's own liability for failure to investigate cause a tremendous amount of confusion and stress among mental health practitioners. Yet the hallmark of a profession, as noted, is self-regulation. If professionals do not effectively discharge this duty to self-regulate, outside bodies such as government agencies or the courts will be more likely to do it for us. On the other hand, it is important to all professionals to achieve a certain degree of professional autonomy and to trust their own ability to make decisions. The development of a vigilante society policing itself is distasteful to all conscientious professionals. Thus, a reasonable balance is needed. This chapter deals with issues involved in confronting potentially unethical or potentially impaired colleagues. It also describes some of the ways in which typical professional ethics committees function and the issues that arise when one is oneself the subject of an investigation or allocation.

In essence, these notions underlie the concept of a profession. Members of a profession are generally autonomous; they are not supervised or directed by other professions. Members of a profession are therefore self-monitoring; they take on the obligation to insure that all who belong to the profession adhere to some common standards. These notions thus imply that, whether one is on the receiving or the giving end of professional peer scrutiny, one has the obligation to treat colleagues (as well as members of related professions) responsibly.

THE UNETHICAL PROFESSIONAL

Example 1. In the course of her work in forensics settings, a practitioner becomes aware of a fellow practitioner who has become, in legal slang, a "hired gun," in that he can be reliably counted on to give expert testimony that favors the position of the attorney who retained him. In addition, she believes that her colleague is distorting and misrepresenting relevant facts about the cases in which he is involved.

Example 2. A female client of a therapist tells him about her previous therapist who would hug her at the end of each session and, during the hug, would fondle her breasts. The client questions her new therapist as to whether this was appropriate behavior.

These examples illustrate situations in which a mental health professional becomes aware of the unethical behavior of another professional. The codes of ethics of various mental health disciplines do touch on such situations, but in ways that offer little specific guidance. For instance, the social workers' code of ethics (NASW, 1993) states, "The social worker should take action through appropriate channels against unethical conduct by any other member of the profession" (§V.M.2.). Similarly, psychiatrists "strive to expose those physicians deficient in character or competence, or who engage in fraud or deception" (American Psychiatric Association, 1993, Section 2). According to psychologists' code of conduct (American Psychological Association, 1992), "When psychologists believe that there may have been an ethical violation by another psychologist, they attempt to resolve the issue by bringing it to the attention of that individual, if an informal resolution appears appropriate and the intervention does not violate any confidentiality rights that may be involved" (§8.04).

The codes of the various mental health professions highlight the aspirational obligation of the ethical practitioner to aim his or her efforts toward the benefit of the client. Many difficult situations arise in which it is not the clinician's own performance but the functioning of colleagues that raises the potential of harm. Conversely, it may happen to even the most responsibly and ethically intentioned professional that he or she is the target of an allegation or ethics charge.

In a sense the present chapter focuses on a sort of etiquette of collegial relationships. Many of the issues to be raised are matters of prudence and tact necessary in the upholding of sound ethical standards. Although the obligation to confront colleagues is addressed in a number of ethics codes, the *processes* of so doing are not always entirely clear. In addition, it is frequently not clear what the cost/benefit ratio of such confrontation or consultation might be. The cultural norms against "tattling" or "whistleblowing" are quite strong, and at the same time the failure to deal with errant colleagues is one of the rationales for ever-tighter controls over professionals. Thus it is important to think through in advance and perhaps even rehearse the steps to effective and ethical confrontation of colleagues.

CONFRONTING THE
UNETHICAL PROFESSIONAL

The psychiatrists' code of ethics indicates that "It is ethical, even encouraged, for another psychiatrist to intercede" when a psychiatrist because of mental illness jeopardizes the welfare of patients (American Psychiatric Association, 1993, Section 2.4).

Certainly educating consumers about their rights is an important step in this regard. However, this may be of limited effectiveness in preventing professional difficulties, although it may help in the more rapid detection of problems. Moreover, educating patients or potential patients in ways to detect professional impairment adds a burden to someone who is seeking help that seems inappropriate. Thus we return to the role of the colleague.

Beginning steps in improving the social skill of tactfully confronting colleagues are outlined in a paper by VandenBos and Duthie (1986), in which the authors make several useful suggestions. They advise that it is helpful to approach colleagues in a questioning manner, first ascertaining that one has accurate information. It is important not to presume guilt or innocence in these matters. On the other hand, it is important to be frank about one's concerns and, if one believes that a problem exists, forthright in recommending that the potentially impaired colleague seek help in remedying the difficulties. The field could benefit from case reports of successful use of their approach and inclusion of this issue in graduate and postgraduate training curricula.

Substandard behavior can result from impairment, which may also be considered unethical. The hallmark of unethical behavior is that we believe that individual could have chosen to do otherwise. Instead, he or she chose to act in a way that served the client (or the profession or the society) poorly. Although it is possible that unethical practice is of long duration (e.g., the clinician may never have operated ethically in this context), the distinguishing feature of unethical behavior is that it presumes personal responsibility. The possibility of conscious, deliberate choice is considered to be available to the individual. It is, however, possible, as Keith-Spiegel and Koocher (1985) have pointed out, for unethical behavior to stem from ignorance. Nonetheless we presume that the behavior was not compelled, in the sense that increased knowledge would allow the individual to make a choice. As in the previous case, the solution to the problem primarily lies in providing more information or supervision of professional activities.

It is commonly assumed that a confrontation involves the face-to-face criticism of a colleague for unethical behavior, but this is not necessarily always the case. A "confrontation" may be as gentle and nonthreatening as raising a tactful question about a colleague's behavior or area of responsibility. It may also take a more indirect form, such as reflecting with a colleague (e.g., "You know, I once had a problem like this, and what I did was. . . ."). Of course, the more indirect the approach, the more one must insure that the message was indeed received and not denied. Despite the gentleness of the approach, it remains the case that pointing out possible misconduct on the part of a colleague puts one in a precarious position; one risks alienating the colleague whether or not (perhaps especially if) one is correct about the misconduct. This implies that the practitioner should weigh the potential costs of confrontation against the possible benefits. Potential costs include harm to the collegial relationship and the chance of aggravating the situation in some way, such as if the practitioner retaliates against a client. The major benefit of confrontation is the elimination of harmful or unethical practices. One should also consider the harm that is done to the reputation of the profession if confrontation is avoided and the harmful practices continue. If slight but damaging ethical misdeeds are left unchallenged, tolerance of collegial misconduct rapidly leads to perceptions among laypersons that a profession is cynically self-serving. On the other hand, constant chiding from one's colleagues can lead to a sort of competition among professionals to point out each other's wrongdoing. This state of affairs can escalate into avoidable charges being filed with the state association's or the national association's ethics committees regarding colleagues' behavior (D. Mills, personal communication, 1984).

It is also important to note that the presumption of innocence may be as important as tactfulness in confronting colleagues. Many professionals commit ethical violations out of ignorance rather than "willful disregard" of ethical standards (Keith-Spiegel, 1977). In addition, often the confronting professional has only indirect evidence of the substandard conduct.

What, then, is the appropriate course of action? As Vanden-Bos and Duthie (1986) suggest, when aware of evidence that may indicate that a colleague is behaving unethically, one should first ascertain the facts. Thus, an informal inquiry might be in order.

At the same time, ordinary tact would dictate that one not pursue questions in an insensitive or hostile fashion. However, not infrequently a colleague will react defensively to an inquiry. If the suspected misdeed is serious enough, this requires that one report concerns to the appropriate regulatory group (i.e., licensing board or ethics committee). Such an action will not endear one to a colleague whose actions are questioned, and it is certainly advisable to first consider the alternatives. A possible course of action might involve an attempt to consult with respected colleagues. Following this, if consultation supports one's views, an attempt at confrontation; if confrontation fails or is inappropriate, a report to the ethics committee or licensing board might be in order.

One issue to keep in mind is the confidentiality of the client; this is particularly a problem when one's current client reveals improper behavior by a previous therapist. Clearly the therapist cannot respond to your inquiry without breaching confidentiality, nor can the client be identified to the questioned therapist without the client's permission. These sorts of cases are probably best handled by encouraging the client to file a complaint directly. However, this raises problems too, because the client will then have to confront his or her previous therapist. If the client chooses not to do this, despite feelings of frustration and anger, there is nothing further that the ethical therapist can do.

Practitioners in more vulnerable positions, such as trainees or students who are having difficulty with the actions of their superiors, are a special case. Such individuals may fear they could harm their chances for completing training if they come forward with questions about their supervisors' behavior. For psychologists, there is a "statute of limitations" that is somewhat of a protection. That is, the psychologist who is in a training position who wishes to file an ethics charge has a period of 3 years from the date at which the training status is terminated in which the charge can be filed.

A final consideration concerning confrontation is that of separating one's emotional reactions from one's professional reactions. It is easy to rationalize the misconduct of one's friends and easy to judge too harshly the conduct of one's enemies. Again, weighing the consequences of confrontation against the consequences of

the misdeed continuing is essential in arriving at a balanced conclusion. Evaluating the alternatives to direct confrontation when
one is considering the actions of a disliked colleague, and considering the usefulness of a gentle inquiry when reviewing the actions
of a liked colleague, are both appropriate steps.

One of the ethical difficulties in professional life with colleagues who have different skills is not giving them work or
teaching them activities which they are not qualified to provide.
For example, the psychiatrists' code of ethics with specific reference to psychologists states that psychiatrists do not delegate any
matter requiring the exercise of professional medical judgment.
This could be a little inflammatory. On the other hand, the psychologists' code indicates that psychologists do not promote the
use of psychological assessment techniques by unqualified persons.
Marriage and family therapists are urged to be certain that the
qualifications of persons in their employ are represented in a manner that is not false, misleading, or deceptive. Similarly social
workers are obligated to prevent the unauthorized or unqualified
practice of social work.

CONFRONTING THE POSSIBLY IMPAIRED PROFESSIONAL

Drug and alcohol abuse, psychological disorders, burnout, and
other impairments affect mental health professionals just as they
do the general public (VandenBos & Duthie, 1986). Often the
impaired or distressed* professional's colleagues will be in the
best position to confront the difficulties. It is useful to remember
that impaired professionals are frequently skillful at denying and
rationalizing their difficulties. The limited literature available on
this topic (e.g., Freudenberger, 1982; Norcross & Prochaska, 1983;
VandenBos & Duthie, 1986) suggests that mental health professionals have difficulty admitting that they need help and often
believe that they are simply situationally troubled.

---

*Many experts distinguish between *impaired* professionals, who have disorders that harm their
work, and *distressed* professionals, who are emotionally upset but who maintain an adequate
level of work (VandenBos & Duthie, 1986).

It is often difficult for distressed professionals to find other sources of help. Especially when they reach the senior ranks of the mental health professions, finding a therapist who can be trusted and respected may be difficult. A frequent rationale for avoiding confrontation - "I'm sure he realizes that he has a problem and is doing something about it" - is thus unlikely to be a valid reason for inaction. Further, the notion that the disorder may be time-limited is not valid in all cases. When we deal with noncolleagues, we typically claim that treatment can help to restore efficient functioning. Presumably we should apply the same expectations to ourselves.

Confrontation in the case of an impaired practitioner is likely to be quite similar to the process noted previously. That is, questioning, empathizing, and gentle reminders may be of considerable help in bringing the issue to light, especially when one has a trusting relationship with the colleague. On the other hand, sometimes one encounters distressed professionals with whom one does not have a trusting relationship. Again, one attempts to use clinical skills and tact to bring the matter to the colleague's attention. If these efforts are met with defensiveness and hostility, it may be appropriate to bring the matter to the attention of a regulatory body. It is also important that the responsible practitioner be aware of resources for the distressed professional. For example, physicians in many states as well as the American Medical Association nationally have developed model programs and model statutes for "disabled doctors" (Laliotis & Grayson, 1985). In addition, psychologists' developing network, *Psychologists Helping Psychologists*, is another resource both for impaired colleagues and for ideas concerning program development. Many state professional associations now operate "colleague assistance" programs for drug- or alcohol-abusing professionals in recovery.

BEING CONFRONTED

Even the best intentioned professional may, for good or poor reasons, find himself or herself confronted by a colleague because of concerns about professional behavior. From an ethical perspective, it is apparent that the practitioner being confronted should consider objectively the nature of the concern being expressed. It is probably obvious to any competent, mature practitioner that it is best to view challenges as opportunities to learn rather than occasions to counterattack. Nonetheless, a few obvious issues in this domain are probably worth emphasizing. Given the natural human tendency to be angry and defensive in such situations, it is likely that one's first response will be to disqualify the message or the messenger in some way, for instance, "How dare he tell me that I have done anything wrong? He's the most arrogant therapist I've ever seen," or "She doesn't know good therapy when she sees it." The person being confronted may be tempted to question the motives of the confronting practitioner; conceivably, the motives may not be honorable or may reflect some personal agenda such as professional jealousy or personal rivalry. However, the accuser's motives are technically irrelevant, and the confronted practitioner should attempt to set motives aside and deal with the content of the concern. The relevant question is whether there is any substance to the issue raised. The psychologists' code offers the chance to file a countercomplaint of frivolous charges (undoubtedly the other professional ethics bodies would entertain similar charges if merited), but this can only be done after the initial issue has been resolved, so it is best to do this with grace and not inflame one's accuser no matter how much he or she seems to deserve it.

Once the practitioner has succeeded in separating the message from the messenger, the next step is to assess the legitimacy of the concern. Was the action unethical, illegal, unwise, or inappropriate in some other way? In what ways, if any, did it violate the relevant ethical standards? In what ways, if any, did it violate the law? Was a client or other party harmed in any way? Did the reputation of the profession suffer? In answering such questions, as with many discussed in this book, it may be useful to consult a trusted colleague or even to seek advice from the appropriate ethics, professional standards, or licensing committees. It may also be useful to consider the issue in question in terms of some of the dimensions discussed previously in this book. Specifically, could the practitioner defend what he or she did to a group of peers? In a similar situation, would the practitioner do the same thing again and recommend that others do the same?

If the result of these deliberations is that the practitioner feels that no violation was committed, then he or she may wish to report back to the individual who expressed the concern, stating the process that was employed and the reasons for the decision that was made. If, on the other hand, the practitioner decides that the action in question was in fact inappropriate, then corrective steps should be determined. If a client was harmed, steps must be taken to rectify the harm. There should also be steps taken to assure that the behavior will never recur. Again, it may be desirable to notify the confronting practitioner of what conclusions were drawn and what remedial steps were taken. Certainly one should document the actions one took in case further accusations emerge. If the questioned actions are indeed fairly serious, it may be better to submit the problem to the local or national ethics committee for resolution. This is recommended because (a) ethics committees do have as part of their charge an educative function so that they may help a practitioner learn what caused the problem (note the difference between ethics committees and licensing boards, which have the charge to protect the public - they ordinarily are not good sources for advisory opinions); and (b) having the matter resolved formally will prevent an informal resolution being followed by formal charges. It is certainly not unknown for well-meaning therapists to attempt an "informal" resolution that involves recontacting an upset and volatile ex-client who then becomes even more upset by the contact and subsequently files formal charges.

DEALING WITH ETHICS COMMITTEES

No practitioner wants to be asked to respond to an ethics committee to explain his or her activities, but many practitioners find themselves in such a situation. Regardless of whether or not the practitioner considers such a request appropriate, it is wise to deal in advance with issues of defensiveness, hostility, and the like. Whenever possible, it is helpful to think of ethics committees as composed of one's colleagues, rather than being composed of inquisitors. It is helpful to view the process as potentially improving the quality of one's professional work, rather than to think of it as a trial in which one side is right and the other wrong. These are idealistic notions, of course; because ethics committee members are human, they sometimes can become overly punitive. And because practitioners questioned about ethics matters are also human, they may become overly defensive and hostile. Nonetheless, a focus on the ultimate point of the enterprise - the well-being of clients - may help to reduce the defensiveness on both sides. Defensiveness by the "complainee" can be particularly damaging to even an innocent professional; it will cause the committee to become suspicious.

Many state ethics committees subscribe to the rules and procedures of the national ethics committee of their parent organization (e.g., many state psychological association ethics committees use the published rules and procedures of the American Psychological Association Ethics Committee; Mills, 1986). It is important to note that for professional association ethics committees, due process is *a* feature but not *the* sole feature in the design of their activities. For example, it is a key feature of due process that a "defendant" be permitted to confront the accuser. For reasons of protecting the (presumably) weaker, complaining client, this is rarely a feature of ethics committees' procedure in hearing charges. Psychologists, for example, frequently conduct the investigation entirely on paper; psychiatrists often have both parties present. Conversely, it is sometimes not obvious to observers why ethics committees keep so much of their activities confidential; shouldn't the profession at large, or consumers for that matter, know who has been charged with what? Despite these pressures, ethics committees exist to change professionals' appropriate practices and not necessarily to punish the guilty.

There have been cases brought to ethics committees by aggrieved clients after they had been contacted by guilty therapists who attempted to make restitution for their previous misbehavior. In some of these cases, these contacts reopened the wounds and resulted in the filing of formal charges regardless.

RELATED AREAS

Although we do not advocate mental health professionals becoming vigilantes concerning the behavior of colleagues in allied disciplines, it is nonetheless true that the various disciplines are linked together in important ways. Among them is the issue of the public's trust in mental health professionals. Thus, in addition to the obligation to be aware of the special contributions of each of the mental health disciplines (which allows one to make sensible referrals), there is the issue of awareness of the ethical codes by which they practice. With regard to interprofessional relationships, a psychologist's code of ethics indicates that psychologists "cooperate with other professionals in order to serve their patients or clients effectively and appropriately" (American Psychological Association, 1992, §1.20b). In addition, referral practices must be consistent with law.

Psychiatrists, probably because of the long medical tradition (now defunct) of treating other physicians at no charge, known as professional courtesy, have excluded it in their ethics code. "Professional courtesy may lead to poor psychiatric care for physicians and their families because of embarrassment over the lack of a complete give and take contract" (American Psychiatric Association, §6.1).

Appendices A to D (pp. 193-258) contain the ethical codes of psychiatry, psychology, social work, and marriage and family therapy; the reader is encouraged to review them and note points of similarity and differences with his or her own profession's code. There may be times when a professional will have to deal with the misconduct of a practitioner of another discipline. In addition to some familiarity with the codes of other disciplines, the professional should have at least enough familiarity with the regulatory bodies of other disciplines to know how to institute disciplinary proceedings.

Chapter 10

Ethical Issues
in Record Keeping

Despite significant professional disagreements about the extent and desirability of record keeping, it has become clear that records in some form are essential to the responsible practice of the mental health professions. The mental health record serves several crucial functions: First, records are clinical tools, for example, reminding the clinician of important themes and perceptions related to the case, or providing information needed by colleagues who may subsequently become involved with the case; second, records can serve as legal documents in such circumstances as malpractice actions, divorce proceedings, or child custody cases; and third, insurance companies and other third parties may rely on clinicians' records to document the amount, nature, and duration of services rendered.

Perhaps because of disputes about the need for keeping records, the codified ethical standards of the various mental health professions offer little in the way of specific guidelines for record keeping (cf. *General Guidelines for Providers of Psychological Services*, American Psychological Association, 1987). However, with or without specific standards, clinicians who practice responsibly must attend to a number of ethical concerns. Records can "speak" for the clinician or the patient; they can be used to document the provision of competent, responsible service; they can be used (or abused) to compromise the client's rights of confidentiality; and they can, when released to others, raise questions of patients' autonomy and informed consent. The importance of accurate records cannot be underestimated (Suisson, VandeCreek, & Knapp, 1987). Many ethical and competent therapists have been found negligent because they did not maintain adequate records. This chapter is devoted to the ethical dimensions of these and related issues raised in the course of record keeping. The first section suggests what might constitute relevant (and irrelevant) aspects of a client's chart. Second, we review some of the situations in which clinical information is released. Third, some general considerations in maintaining the security of records are described.

WHAT SHOULD BE
INCLUDED IN RECORDS

A wide range of record-keeping practices exists among clinicians: from avoidance of the practice to the keeping of almost verbatim accounts. At the one extreme, clinicians contend that it is inappropriate to keep records at all. This position stems from one of two ideas: that record keeping (or at least note taking) disrupts the "here and now" nature of therapy; or that record keeping (or the absence of records) provides protection against subpoena. At the other end of the spectrum are those clinicians who painstakingly record virtually every word the client says, making no effort to separate the important from the trivial. From an ethical perspective, both positions pose problems. Certainly without records or notes there is nothing to be released, but at the same time there is no way to document competent service or to remind yourself of concerns discussed with the client. On the other hand, although including everything in the chart obviously provides extensive documentation, it also increases the amount of client information that is revealed if the records are subpoenaed. It may even decrease the usefulness of the information to subsequent therapists, inasmuch as they may be reluctant to read a massive transcript.

In determining what should be included in charts, the clinician should consider his or her potential "audiences": for whom is the chart being written? Described on the next page are the typical audiences for which the clinician writes, including the types of information that each audience requires.

1. *The clinician himself or herself, and other practitioners.* Records should obviously be a resource to the clinician himself or herself. Patients come and go from treatment, and treatment is interrupted by illness, travel, and other external forces. It is unlikely that the clinician will have perfect recall of all relevant themes and issues important in treatment, which makes clinical notes necessary. In addition, patients move, need referrals to other practitioners with different specialties, or resume treatment with a different therapist after termination. These cases, too, require adequate records to serve the client properly. Indeed, the clinician should consider what information would prove useful if another clinician had to take over the case because of the initial therapist's sudden demise or incapacity. Further, if at some time in the future the client again seeks treatment, good records may make more efficient the subsequent assessment or treatment-planning process.

2. *The patient.* Patients themselves sometimes wish to review their charts (this issue is discussed in more detail later in this chapter) and typically have the right to do so. Although the clinical issues behind a request to review the record should be thoroughly explored, it is good clinical practice to write one's notes in such a way that one would not be troubled unduly if the client himself or herself were to read them. Clients often are curious about what issues they discussed at earlier points in treatment, they sometimes suffer memory lapses about what "homework" the therapist assigned to them, and sometimes transference reactions generate suspicion about what the therapist is writing about them.

3. *Third-party payers.* Third-party payers routinely investigate what disorder is being treated to determine whether it is covered under the terms of the policy or contract. Insurance providers also want to know that services have

actually been provided and that the type of services provided are considered appropriate. The clinical record is a typical means of documenting these factors. Although insurance carriers and, increasingly, managed care companies ask for very detailed, sensitive information, such information should not normally be volunteered, and the rationale for needing it should be questioned. For this reason, it is generally wise to keep financial records separate from clinical records in order to minimize the broadcasting of confidential information. A complete record, for insurance purposes, should not typically need to include more than date of service, type of service, charges and payments, and the diagnosis of the disorder treated.

4. *The legal system* (courts and attorneys). As noted earlier, charts may be subpoenaed as part of court proceedings. Such actions include malpractice suits against the therapist, criminal actions against the client, or some form of civil action such as a divorce or custody suit. As a defense against a malpractice suit, it is important that records reflect that the clinician has been responsible in conceptualizing the case and devising a treatment plan. Issues of suicide risk and the potential for physical aggressiveness should be included (even if only to note that they have been ruled out), so that it is clear from the chart that these things have not simply been overlooked (Cohen, 1979). Also, if the client demonstrates any symptomatology that may have a medical component, such as depression or thought disorder, the records should document that these factors have been considered as well.

In summary, it is our recommendation that records be written with the potential audiences in mind and that only information necessary to meet such needs be included in a client's chart. It is assumed that chart notes will be written in a professional, objective, and nonpejorative manner. It is critical that speculations be clearly defined as such and that caution be exercised in writing down allegations or hunches. Once something is included in a chart, it becomes archival and may be given more importance than it merits. Because of this potential, some responsible practitioners routinely review their charts, eliminating speculations and other obsolete material.

RELEASING RECORDS

There are a number of situations in which clinicians may be called upon to release their records or information contained in them. Below are listed the most common of these situations along with some of the ethical issues the clinician should consider.

RESPONDING TO SIGNED
RELEASES OF INFORMATION

There are numerous occasions on which the clinician is given permission by the client to release information. There are not necessarily any ethical problems with releasing information if the client has signed an appropriate release of information form that includes the name of the requesting organization, the name and signature of the client, the purpose of the release, the extent of the information released, and the date on which the release expires or can be revoked (Kinzie, Holmes, & Arent, 1985). However, certain factors in this process may have ethical implications. For one, it may be wise for the clinician to consider whether the client was able to give voluntary informed consent for the release. Kinzie et al. (1985) surveyed 32 patients who released all or part of their psychiatric records; 81% of these patients felt that release of the information was mandatory in order to continue to receive medical, financial, or other help. This finding raises the question of whether or not releases of information are truly voluntary. If, for instance, refusing to sign a release of information form would result in an insurance company's refusal to pay the bill, then the client has been more or less coerced into giving permission to release information, regardless of fears about the risk to which they are exposed. Although it should not be expected that the clinician will absorb the loss if the client refuses to give permission to release information, the clinician should do whatever is possible to broaden the client's alternatives. The clinician may release only limited summaries (admittedly there is some cost to the therapist in preparing these separately from the clinical record), may attempt to change the third party's policy of demanding detailed information, or may discuss with the client (hopefully in advance) the types of information that could be requested and who is likely to have access to that information. Again, in light of the suggestions made earlier in this chapter, it is important to release only that information necessary for the purposes at hand. It is also important to note that the *clinician's* record-keeping policies are irrelevant to the insurance carrier's requests. That is, even if the practitioner keeps no records at all, the third-party payor may insist on detailed treatment information before authorizing payment. Discussion of the merits of continuing to deal with such a carrier are beyond the scope of this chapter.

If information is being released for legal purposes, the client should be informed that once permission is given, he or she is not usually able to restrict what is released. Clients involved in divorce actions, for instance, might understandably wish to release only that information which casts them in a positive light; they must be made aware that if they give permission to have information released for a certain purpose, all information that bears on that purpose is then accessible. A similar issue is found in disability insurance claims in which job stress is made an issue; the employee attempting to claim benefits may not be able to restrict the extent of information released.

Another issue the clinician must keep in mind when responding to a written release of information is that he or she is empowered to release information only about the person or persons who sign the release. For example, if a couple is seen in conjoint therapy and then at some later point the clinician receives a release of information form signed by only one of the partners, he or she is able only to release information about that one individual. The clinician would be wise to anticipate such an occurrence and keep charts in ways that would allow for the subsequent extraction of information on any individual client. Alternatively, the therapist might stipulate to the couple beforehand that records will be released only if both agree. If there is concern that a particularly litigious client will challenge such a policy, the practitioner should get a legal review of his or her informed consent statement.

A final point about responding to releases of information relates to dealing with requests for information from other professionals. Good client care requires that a clinician seek information about a client's previous treatment. In fact, *Jablonski v. United States* (1983) held, in part, that a clinician was liable for not obtaining previous records. Based on this, it is incumbent on responsible therapists to obtain prior records. Although most therapists who have made such requests have found a very low rate of response, it bears mentioning here that it is extremely inconsiderate to fellow professionals not to respond promptly to requests for information.

RESPONDING TO SUBPOENAS

Clinicians who are not familiar with the legal system can be intimidated when receiving a subpoena. It is as if they feel a document that looks so official and formal must override the client's right to confidentiality. As R. L. Schwitzgebel and R. K. Schwitzgebel (1980) have pointed out, however, there are different kinds of subpoenas, and not all of them demand the immediate release of records. Attorneys who have no legitimate right to the records will sometimes bluster and threaten, hoping that the clinician will be sufficiently intimidated to release the information. Clinicians who are not confident of their legal ground in this area or who have little familiarity with the subpoena process should get legal advice before turning over records. In addition, clients' attorneys should be consulted as well. As R. L. Schwitzgebel and R. K. Schwitzgebel (1980) have suggested, the best course of action when faced with a subpoena is to do nothing until one is sure of the appropriate course of action. Such a delay will not usually get a practitioner into trouble, but hasty and improper release of records might do so.

ALLOWING CLIENTS ACCESS
TO THEIR OWN CHARTS

There is considerable difference of opinion regarding the extent to which a client should have access to his or her own records. Roth, Wolford, and Meisel (1980) have summarized the various arguments about this. Reasons cited to prohibit a client's access to charts include the assertion that medical records are often unintelligible to the layperson, that revelation of certain information could be detrimental, and that records may contain references to or information from other individuals who could be harmed by such release. Arguments in favor of increased access to records include issues of freedom of information, informed consent in the client's release of records, and other matters of client autonomy.

From a legal perspective, it has typically been held that clinicians have considerable discretion in terms of whether or not to allow clients access to their records (Roth et al., 1980). If, in the clinician's judgment, seeing the records would be harmful to a client or would violate the confidentiality of a third person, a request to review the records can be denied, but the client does have the right to choose a professional to represent him or her and review the record (Roth et al., 1980). Private practitioners have somewhat more latitude on this issue than those in public service. Federal freedom-of-information regulations, as well as the Family Education and Right to Privacy Act (FERPA, or the "Buckley Amendment," PL 93-380, 1974) mandate records disclosure policies for agencies receiving federal funding. In other circumstances, state statutes prevail, and the practitioner would be well advised to review statutes of the states in which he or she practices.

From an ethical viewpoint, the question of whether or not to allow a client access to his or her records contains elements of the autonomy-paternalism conflict discussed earlier. If the clinician's decision were based solely on sustaining client autonomy, then the client would have total access to his or her records. If the decision were based completely on paternalism, then the client would justifiably be denied access to the records, because the clinician would be empowered to act in the client's best interests, and client input would be unnecessary. From this perspective, client access to the chart would be unwise because it might limit the practitioner's power of discretion. In light of our previous discussion of the autonomy-paternalism question, we believe that autonomy should be the overriding principle; clients should have access to information in their charts unless there is a justifiable reason to deny such access.

Clients' requests to view their records are not common, but the clinician would still be wise to anticipate such an eventuality. Records should be kept in a way that reflects solid professional judgment and respect for the client. Obviously, pejorative statements should be avoided.

To summarize, the clinician does have a right to deny access to a chart if he or she feels that something contained in it would be damaging to the client or would violate a third party's rights. Nonetheless, he or she should be ready to deal with the client's request in a therapeutic way that still safeguards client rights. Examples of such procedures include presenting a verbal summary of the information, or offering to review the records with another professional of the client's choosing. It is of course necessary to thoroughly probe the clinical issues that are emerging in such requests, and it is frequently not necessary to accede literally to the request to turn over records to the client (e.g., portions of the chart may be read to the patient rather than handing him or her the entire document).

GENERAL CONSIDERATIONS
REGARDING THE
SECURING OF RECORDS

We assume that all practitioners are aware of their obligation to maintain their records in a way that protects the client's confidentiality. However, it is easy to get so accustomed to one's own routine that breaches of the confidentiality of records can occur in subtle and unexpected ways. Consider the illustration of a receptionist in a therapist's office who was discovered reading records of one of the clients, an attorney whom the receptionist was considering retaining. She was very open in explaining that she wanted to see whether the man could be trusted. She was a new receptionist, and the process of her training regarding the use of records was obviously lacking.

As another example, it is very easy to get into the habit of leaving client records on one's desk, making them accessible to other clients or office visitors. Such potential breaches are very numerous and, as noted, can occur even within the most responsible of record-keeping systems.

One area in which security of information is often compromised involves the telephone. Answering services should be carefully assessed to insure that they understand proper procedure for taking and securing messages. Likewise, telephone machines should be carefully monitored, and care should be taken to insure that no one but appropriate staff can hear incoming messages.

We recommend that practitioners periodically review their own behavior and their office practices with an eye toward such potential breaches. Clerical and other nonclinical staff should be included in this review; because nonclinical staff are not bound by the same ethical codes nor trained in appropriate procedures, careful orientation and supervision of them is necessary. Despite this difference in background, the practitioner bears the ultimate responsibility for the actions of his or her staff. Staff should be thoroughly trained in the relevant issues and reminded of their obligations to safeguard confidentiality. The practitioner might want to review or discuss record-keeping practices with a colleague in order to jointly benefit from fresh perspectives. An outsider may be able to point out things that the clinician, because of his or her familiarity with the routine, might not see.

DISPOSAL OF RECORDS

For both practical and ethical reasons, the practitioner at some point may need to destroy records which are no longer relevant or useful. There are two important considerations in this regard: when to dispose of the records and how to do so. In terms of the first of these concerns, a number of factors need to be kept in mind. The practitioner needs to maintain records as long as there is a chance that they will be needed. As Keith-Spiegel and Koocher (1985) have pointed out, records may be needed for financial reasons (e.g., to serve as documentation for an IRS audit) or they may be needed to provide for continuity of care should a client again enter into treatment. Further, legal situations may arise which may make the details of treatment relevant at a later date.

Despite the obligation not to dispose of records prematurely, the length of time they should be kept is by no means clear. State and federal statutes vary as to the minimum length of time records should be kept. Keith-Spiegel and Koocher (1985) recommend keeping records at least 7 years from the termination of treatment, even if state statutes specify a shorter time period. This corresponds with the length of time that the IRS can audit a tax return. In the *Specialty Guidelines for the Delivery of Services by Clinical Psychologists* (American Psychological Association, 1981), it is recommended that the full record be retained intact for 3 years after completion of planned services or after the last date of contact with the consumer (whichever is later), and that the full record or a summary of the record be maintained for an additional 12 years. The record may be entirely disposed of no sooner than 15 years after completion of planned services or after the date of the last contact, whichever is later.

The practitioner may of course opt to keep records forever. Because relevant guidelines specify minimum time periods, such a course of action may be justified. However, this places other demands on the practitioner. Extremely old information may have become obsolete or irrelevant. Should this information be obtained by the legal system or employers, it may serve as the basis of inappropriate decisions. This concern places extra demands on the practitioner to secure records. Further, as will be discussed below, a practitioner who opts to keep records indefinitely should formulate plans for the disposition of the records in the event of death or severe disability.

As mentioned, in addition to the question of when to dispose of records, there is also the question of how to do so. It is important that they be disposed of in a safe, effective manner. Throwing confidential information in the trash is not adequate. A psychiatrist of our acquaintance was dismayed when he came to work one morning and found a draft of a psychiatric evaluation he had written lying on the sidewalk in front of his office door. He had thrown it in the garbage, the custodians had placed it in the dumpster, and the wind had blown it out. Any information with clients' names should be shredded (hopefully this will still allow the discharge of the ethical duty to recycle).

The psychologists' code of ethics mandates that psychologists must plan in advance so that the confidentiality of records is maintained regardless of whether the psychologist abruptly leaves the practice, becomes incapacitated, or dies. Also, psychologists recognize that records and data must remain available to clients directly in some cases (e.g., custody evaluation reports). Because of a number of ethics complaints that involved withholding of records for nonpayment of fees, the psychologists' code explicitly prohibits linking these two activities. It is called "holding records hostage" and in the revised code it is now considered unethical.

The psychiatrists' code recognizes that the records must be "protected with extreme care" (American Psychiatric Association, 1993, §4.1). No other guidance is given. The social workers' code of ethics mandates that social workers should avoid clients' reasonable access to any official social work records concerning them although any confidences of others contained in those records must be protected. Marriage and family therapists are obligated to "store or dispose of client records in ways that maintain confidentiality" (AAMFT, 1991, §2.3).

Chapter 11

The Financial Side of Practice: Billing, Collecting, and Other Money Matters

Despite the helping nature of the mental health professions, it is not unethical for clinicians to want to profit financially in their practices, nor is it inherently unethical to desire a relatively high income. However, because the practitioner's economic survival depends on payment from clients and third-party sources, decision making on financial issues can easily be influenced by less than purely ethical motives. In a subtle way, financial considerations may lead the practitioner to make ethically unjustifiable decisions, perhaps even without awareness that money motivates them. Conversely, as mental health practice becomes more commercial, practitioners who would prefer not to think about the monetary aspects of what they do may find themselves inadvertently putting themselves or their clients in difficult situations.

The purpose of this chapter is to point out some of the more commonly observed ethical problems connected with the financial aspects of clinical practice. Whenever possible, we discuss practical solutions to the problems raised. In so doing, we are attempting to help providers become more comfortable with the fact that they are indeed *selling* their services; we also hope to demonstrate that a clinician can practice at a high level ethically and still survive financially, or as the old phrase has it, "do good and still do well."

The present chapter first covers potential ethical problems in charging and collecting fees from clients. Then insurance-related matters are discussed. The final section briefly discusses fee-splitting.

BILLING AND
COLLECTING FROM CLIENTS

There are a number of financial matters that a practitioner must consider in dealing with clients. Among these are providing information about financial matters, collecting on bad debts, and considering whether to exchange professional services for services or goods from clients. In the following sections, each of these will be discussed.

PROVIDING INFORMATION
ABOUT FINANCIAL MATTERS

Practitioners vary considerably in their approaches to fee setting and other financial issues related to their clients. Because of the intimate nature of the therapeutic relationship, many practitioners become extremely uncomfortable with the reality that they are being paid for their time and thus avoid bringing up such "details." These diffident clinicians reveal (or ask for) the minimum information necessary ("Do you have insurance?") or delay discussing fees and financial policies until the last possible minute. Others do not deal directly with money matters, but delegate these tasks to the office staff. Still other practitioners view financial issues as fundamental to clinical practice and make them a part of therapy. Although some latitude in these matters can certainly be appropriate, it is important to remember that the client has a right to know what types of services will be offered, their approximate duration, and the expected costs (Hare-Mustin et al., 1979). It is also helpful to note that a substantial number of ethics complaints are generated by conflict over billing practices. Thus it is not only ethical but also sound business practice to provide appropriate information before exposing clients to a financial obligation they may not understand. The psychiatrists' code of ethics obligates the psychiatrist to be explicit about the provisions of the contract. The psychologists' code mandates that psychologists reach an agreement with consumers or payors as early as possible regarding fees and billing arrangements. Marriage and family therapists make "reasonably understandable" financial arrangements that "conform to accepted professional practices" (AAMFT, 1991, §7). They do not charge excessive fees, they disclose their fees at the beginning of services, and they accurately represent the services provided. Social workers are obligated to set fees that are "fair, reasonable, considerate, and commensurate with the service performed and with due regard for the clients' ability to pay" (NASW, 1993, §II.I.).

The nature of the therapeutic relationship makes this process different from the negotiations that would precede remodeling a kitchen or buying a car; some clinicians do not provide sufficient financial information because they have not developed a way of doing so that fits well with the flow of therapy. A client typically comes in for therapy highly distressed and anxious to begin. Thus to start off with a detailed description of financial and other matters necessary for informed consent may seem clumsy and inappropriate. Nonetheless, prospective clients need the financial facts, perhaps especially so if they are highly distressed and perhaps vulnerable to becoming dependent on the therapist. As discussed in Chapter 5, a written handout covering all necessary information may be given to the client before the session. The clinician may simply ask if the handout was read and if there were any questions, and then (assuming that the client is competent to make such decisions) the clinician may obtain a signature consenting to the conditions outlined before the session begins. The information should include provisions for what steps will be taken if fees are not paid.

COLLECTING ON BAD DEBTS

Mental health practitioners have another limitation not shared with other professionals who charge and collect fees - their options in collecting on bad debts. Faustman (1982) has pointed out that even turning the name and address of a client over to a collection agency can be a breach of confidentiality and, as such, may be prohibited unless specific consent has been provided by the client. This, however, has been liberalized in the current *Ethical Principles of Psychologists and Code of Conduct* (American Psychological Association, 1992, §1.25). For this reason we recommend that before treatment begins, the client be informed how bad debts will be collected and be asked to give written permission or acknowledgment that bad debts will be turned over to a collection agency or attorney. If indeed an overdue account accumulates (frequently after the client leaves therapy), the debtor should be warned with sufficient time to pay the debt before a collection agency is contacted.

Cohen (1979) found that fee disputes served as a stimulus for numerous legal actions against psychologists. Clients who leave therapy dissatisfied may respond to aggressive fee collection attempts by instituting malpractice suits against their therapists. Although this is more an issue of prudence than specifically an ethical concern, it is something clinicians would be advised to consider when deciding what to do with bad debts.

For both ethical and practical reasons, it would seem that the best solution to collecting on bad debts would be not to allow them to develop in the first place. Faustman (1982) suggests the following:

1. Expect payment at the time of service.
2. Use charge cards, filling out receipts in ways that do not reveal the therapeutic nature of the service.
3. Negotiate extended payment plans with clients.

B. E. Bennett et al. (1990) also suggest a series of steps the prudent therapist should take to avoid later problems with financial issues, under the heading "running a professional office."

TRADING SERVICES OR GOODS

One creative solution to a client's inability to pay for therapy might seem to be barter or trade, either of goods or of services. The therapist could, for example, provide psychotherapy in exchange for plumbing work. However, such arrangements are almost universally seen as unacceptable, at least among psychologists (Haas et al., 1986; Hall & Hare-Mustin, 1983). Part of the reason for this is that such arrangements are likely to create a problematic dual relationship between the practitioner and the client. It is not difficult to anticipate some of the other problems that these practices would lead to, such as the difficulty in trying to equate the value of the services offered, what would happen if one or the other party was dissatisfied with the service, and so on.

The practice of bartering or trading *goods*, rather than services, is not so clear-cut from an ethical perspective (Hall & Hare-Mustin, 1983) because it is theoretically possible to trade therapeutic services for artwork or other material items without creating the inherent dual relationship problems that occur with trading services. At the very least, however, if a clinician is considering providing therapy in exchange for some object of value, there should be a fair way of assessing the market value of the object, and this value should be agreed upon in advance. However, the clinician is cautioned that although such arrangements may make clinical services accessible to more individuals, they may also complicate the nature of the relationship if one or the other party is dissatisfied with the value received.

In summary, though it is not inherently unethical to engage in bartering goods or services, it appears to us that the wise or prudent practitioner should avoid it in most if not all cases. The standard for psychologists (American Psychological Association, 1992) is that "Psychologists ordinarily refrain from accepting goods, services, or other nonmonetary remuneration from patients or clients in return for psychological services because such arrangements create inherent potential for conflicts, exploitation, and distortion of the professional relationship. A psychologist may participate in bartering *only* if (1) it is not clinically contraindicated, *and* (2) the relationship is not exploitative" (§1.18). This seems an appropriate guideline for all mental health professions.

ISSUES RELATED TO
THIRD-PARTY PAYORS

The practitioner's dependence on insurance companies can lead to a number of practices that are ethically ill-advised. Some of the more troublesome are described as follows.

BILLABLE DIAGNOSES
("UP-CODING" OR "DOWN-CODING")

Insurance policies do not typically cover all diagnostic categories. Usually, if the client's only diagnosis is a V-Code (American Psychiatric Association, 1994), such as parent-child or marital problems, insurance policies will not cover the service. This fact, combined with the client's need for insurance coverage to help defray the costs of treatment, can lead to the practice of giving the client a "billable" diagnosis, even if such a diagnosis is not the most accurate.

In justifying this behavior, a clinician could come up with a number of explanations that are apparently ethical. It could be asserted, for example, that this is the only way for a client to get the help that he or she desperately needs, making inaccurate diagnosis the lesser of two ethical evils. In response to this, it should be noted that a practitioner who takes such an action is appropriating another party's funds to achieve what he or she believes to be moral ends. In other words, the practitioner is trying to be ethical with someone else's money. That is, the insurance company is being asked to pay for an intervention that it would not pay for if all the facts were known. As an alternative, if finances are a problem and the client does not have a reimbursable diagnosis, the clinician may wish to consider seeing the client on a sliding scale, an extended pay schedule, or even as part of the clinician's "pro-bono" work. The clinician also exposes himself or herself to significant liability if the client later becomes upset about the diagnosis. This is a serious issue: Certain diagnoses interfere with the ability to obtain life insurance, to obtain security clearances, and to get later reinsurance (they are then considered "pre-existing conditions"). These issues are not simple, and, aside from the issues of honesty and paternalism involved, there is an issue of short-term versus long-term benefit to the client. The best policy, as the cliché says, is honesty. Working to change the insurance regulations or the cultural stigma around "mental illness" are long range but the only ethical alternatives.

From a "financial survival" perspective, the clinician can take certain steps to minimize the economic impact he or she might experience if an insurance company refuses to reimburse for treatment of an accurately diagnosed disorder. First, the clinician should not guarantee insurance coverage. It should be clear at the start that paying the bill is the responsibility of the client, even if the therapist will actively participate in filling out insurance forms.

Such a stance may be resisted by clients who would prefer that the clinician bill the insurance company, wait until payment is made, and then bill the client for the difference. Alternatively, the clinician may try other strategies that would make his or her policy more palatable. Use of a credit card allows the client to pay a bill on a more leisurely schedule without making the therapist dependent on insurance coverage. Faustman (1982) found that 7.4% of the clinical psychologists he surveyed accepted credit cards. Use of this option might decrease dependence on insurance while being responsive to clients' needs for more time in meeting their obligations. However, one also has an obligation not to induce a client into a treatment relationship which he or she cannot afford to continue through to its proper conclusions. Also, therapists should consider what their policy would be if in the midst of therapy the client suffers a large financial reversal. A sudden referral would be countertherapeutic. How about extended payment? How about reduced fees? What about the resentment this can cause?

WRITING OFF COPAYMENTS

Another insurance-related practice that has ethical implications involves writing off the client's share of the bill and accepting the insurance reimbursement as payment in full. Insurance companies typically pay a certain percentage (often 80%) of the practitioner's customary fee and expect the client to pay the remainder, or copayment (Goodstein, 1983). In the case of financial hardship, waiving the copayment could be of considerable benefit to the client without costing the insurance company any money, because the clinician would absorb the loss. This could be considered an ethical step in certain cases. Insurance companies might consider this inappropriate, but, according to Goodstein, the *occasional* waiving of copayments in cases of financial hardship may not present problems. However, where waiving the copayment becomes a routine practice, it could be viewed as a change in the clinician's usual and customary fee, with insurance companies in effect paying 100% of the clinician's fee. Such a policy could be viewed as deceptive or even fraudulent by an insurance company. Therefore, routinely waiving the copayment would not be considered ethical.

CONFIDENTIALITY IN MAKING CLAIMS

In order to have insurance companies reimburse for therapeutic services, the client must typically sign a release-of-information form that allows the clinician to provide necessary claim information to the insurance company. Such a practice is routine and typically presents no problem ethically. The practitioner should keep certain considerations in mind, however. First, the release form is usually specific in stating that permission is given to provide information necessary for processing the claim. The implication is that care should be taken to release only information necessary for that purpose. Second, it may be wise to have the client consider where the billing information is going to go. Although the clinician is obligated to deal with clinical information in a sensitive and confidential manner, there is no clear-cut similar obligation on insurance company personnel. Therapists should inform themselves of the degree to which insurance carriers share information on diagnoses and services used through the Medical Information Bureau (MIB), a central information bank. It may be helpful for clients to know that they can request copies of their MIB files, although this a somewhat laborious process (MIB, 1993).

The potential for breaches of confidentiality becomes greater in companies which process their own insurance claims, and it would even be possible for a client's claim to be processed by a coworker. It would be appropriate for the clinician to explore such possibilities with the client and, should the client opt not to use insurance, to be flexible in working out alternative payment plans.

RESPONSIBILITY FOR CLIENTS
WHEN INSURANCE BENEFITS END

As people who work in mental health centers and other publicly sponsored agencies are aware, private practitioners sometimes treat clients until the insurance benefits have been exhausted and then refer them to a public agency. It may also be the case that other clients are simply terminated and left to their own devices when their benefits have run out. Ethical practitioners bear a responsibility to their patients which extends beyond insurance benefits. This is not to say that they must, regardless of other considerations, continue seeing clients who can no longer pay. It does mean that at the very least they are obligated to do more than simply tell patients to call a public agency. The clinician might, for example, explore treatment options that would be appropriate given the nature of the client's problem, give the client names of specific practitioners at the agency, or take the responsibility for making sure that the transfer is handled in a constructive manner and (with appropriate permission) provide the receiving therapist with appropriate background information. Clinical issues related to the termination of treatment should be sensitively considered as well.

This is an appropriate context in which to discuss the issue of abandonment. Throughout this book at various junctures we have made reference to the therapist's responsibility to continue treatment and not abandon patients. But what specifically constitutes "abandonment"? VandeCreek, Knapp, and Herzog (1987) have noted that the concept of abandonment has been dealt with more frequently in medical than in psychotherapeutic practice; in the medical arena abandonment refers to the failure to treat or appropriately refer a patient who needs treatment when the provider knows or should have known that continued treatment is necessary. There is no obligation to treat clients who do not need treatment - indeed, there is an ethical obligation in several codes to end professional relationships that are of no benefit to clients

(VandeCreek & Knapp, 1993). However, the therapist and client may differ about the need for continued treatment. When this issue results in disagreement, the therapist must try to make clear his or her reasons for suggesting termination or referral and the client's options for resuming treatment in the future. It is prudent to document this discussion.

FEE-SPLITTING

The term fee-splitting refers to the arrangement in which "part of a sum received for a product or service is returned or paid out because of a prearranged agreement or coercion" (Keith-Spiegel & Koocher, 1985, pp. 158-159). In the simplest case, fee-splitting occurs when a practitioner pays another professional for referrals or receives payment for making referrals. Such practices would be considered unethical under the codes of all mental health disciplines. Fee-splitting is considered unethical primarily because it implies that financial considerations, rather than the individual's welfare, are determining the management of the case. Further, the client is being asked to pay more for a service than is necessary because the amount of money that goes to the referring party represents money paid by the client for which he or she receives no benefit (Keith-Spiegel & Koocher, 1985).

A common example of fee-splitting is the convention of selling one's practice, for instance, when one retires. Although it may appear justifiable to benefit financially from one's accumulated caseload and referral network, it can easily be seen that such a practice fits the definition of fee-splitting in that the practitioner receives remuneration for making referrals to the individual who is buying the caseload. Thus there is a strong likelihood that decisions are dictated not by what is the most beneficial action for the client, but by financial considerations.

Although these examples of fee-splitting are fairly clear-cut, Keith-Spiegel and Koocher (1985) describe some arrangements that are not so obvious. According to those authors, a therapist who hires other therapists, rents them office space, and then collects a percentage of what they collect would be considered to be engaging in fee-splitting, because the percentage that goes to the owner does not benefit the client in any way. It is generally considered justifiable to charge for reasonable office expenses such as telephone and secretarial coverage, supervision and administration expenses, and so on, but Keith-Spiegel and Koocher claim that there should not be charges that are pure profit because it is all too easy in such situations for the financial health of one's group practice to replace the mental health of one's patients as the determining factor in referral patterns. Psychiatry, however, is the only mental health discipline whose code of ethics specifically prohibits fee-splitting arrangements as described previously (American Psychiatric Association, 1993). Psychologists are allowed to split fees as long as they inform the clients fully.

It may be that Keith-Spiegel and Koocher are being too conservative in terms of the types of financial practices they proscribe, especially given the current trends in mental health practice toward profit-making mental health ventures, private psychiatric hospitals, managed care arrangements, and the like. It is becoming more and more difficult to completely avoid financial arrangements that contain at least some elements of fee-splitting, as defined by Keith-Spiegel and Koocher. For example, if a clinician accepts less than his or her customary fee to be considered a preferred provider with a particular insurance company, could this not be considered paying for referrals? Further, if a clinician is a provider who works for a profit-making hospital or clinic, couldn't this also be considered a fee-splitting arrangement in that there is a certain amount of the fee that is profit and thus does not benefit the client?

We believe that the ethical standards of the various mental health disciplines have not kept abreast of these recent developments, and that the practitioner is in something of a bind until they do. Our recommendation is that, until the situation is clarified, practitioners avoid the more direct applications of fee-splitting and the ones which are specifically prohibited by their codes of ethics, such as directly paying or receiving payment for referrals. Beyond that, clinicians should act in ways that protect the well-being of the client and safeguard the client's right to autonomy. For instance, regardless of financial benefits, it would clearly be inappropriate for practitioners to refer a client to a subordinate or coworker if they do not feel confident that the individual is fully competent to handle the presenting problem. Further, it would obviously be inappropriate to recommend treatment that is unnecessarily costly simply because of financial benefit to oneself or one's employees.

In summary, practitioners should be guided by the pertinent ethical codes regarding fee-splitting and should stay current on new developments. They should also be scrupulous in making sure that financial decisions do not endanger the client's welfare or right to competent service. Given the ambiguity of the restrictions regarding fee-splitting, consultation with trusted colleagues or a call to the appropriate committee of one's professional organization may be in order.

Chapter 12

Public Statements:
Advertising, Media
Appearances, and Workshops

Mental health professionals' opinions and ideas are in demand from the public, and it may serve ethical ends to give clinicians more public exposure. For example, a newspaper column on mental health matters may serve an important prevention function in a community, and a call-in advice line may provide immediate, free help to those who would really benefit from it. However, in addition to the possible benefits, there are risks inherent in making public statements.

The mental health practitioner commonly makes public statements (distinct from those made in confidence to patients and colleagues) in several arenas. First, there are professional publications, typically reviewed by peers; second, there are announcements about oneself and one's services made to the public; third, there are requests from the public for advice and information made via the media; and fourth, there are statements made to the press or the media (press conferences, interviews, etc.). Statements made in professional publications are covered by the general standards of scientific and professional writing, and more specifically by the editorial policies of individual journals. The *Publication Manual of the American Psychological Association* (American Psychological Association, 1994) is a good resource in this regard.

Thus, it is on the second and third of these arenas that the present chapter focuses. For the present purposes, the issues will be divided into three topics: (a) issues concerning the provision of information about oneself. These typically concern questions of honesty and responsibility; (b) information concerning general topics in one's area of expertise. This typically raises issues of competence, in addition to those of honesty and responsibility; and (c) information requested by specific persons. This typically adds the issue of conflicts of loyalty to those of honesty, competence, and responsibility.

Although some of these public activities are optional and voluntary, increasingly it is likely that the practitioner will at some point in his or her career be called upon to make public statements. Such statements have the potential for raising or lowering the public's faith in both the person who makes the statement and in the profession represented by that person. Thus there is great concern with such activities by ethics enforcement bodies. If the mental health professions are to retain and enhance their credibility in the public's eyes, statements made by members of those professions must be accurate, honest, useful, and not self-serving.

PUBLIC STATEMENTS ABOUT ONESELF

At the minimum, most practitioners provide telephone listings, professional business cards, and professional announcements as public statements about themselves. In addition, for many practitioners who conduct workshops or publish, there are publishers' announcements, advertisements of workshops, course listings in catalogs, and the like. These sorts of announcements raise two kinds of issues. First there is the issue of "truth in advertising." That is, statements made to the public about oneself and one's services must be designed so as not to mislead or give the wrong impression. There are many ways in which a practitioner can capitalize on the public's lack of information or can use misleading phrases to create a distorted impression. For instance, consider the following statement: "Dr. X did graduate work in clinical psychology at State University and then received his doctorate from Bogus College." One may assume that Dr. X's degree is in clinical psychology, when it could as easily be in anything else. Such a statement is phrased in such a way as to mislead the reader. The phrase ". . . received his doctorate in medieval literature from Bogus College" is much more forthright. Another example might be the use of the term "institute" on one's letterhead when one is the sole provider of services in independent practice. The notion that one is the director of an institute would tend to mislead the naïve consumer into thinking that more resources and prestige are involved than exist in reality. It is more accurate to describe oneself as a solo practitioner if this is in fact the case. This same reasoning underlies the mandatory obligation on psychologists to avoid testimonials from current psychotherapy clients in advertising of services; testimonials are inherently biased and not a scientifically valid means of assessing the effectiveness of services. It can also be argued (as it has been recently by the Federal Trade Commission) that the public's right to know and the professional's right to free trade must be balanced against the risk of misleading the reader. This is the reason that not all clients are prohibited from giving testimonials.

With regard to public statements, the ethics codes of the mental health professions are quite similar. A few interesting differences bear mentioning. The psychologists' ethics code, which in its statements referring to "Advertising and Other Public Statements" (American Psychological Association, 1992), indicates that one's curriculum vitae is also a public statement, as are statements in legal proceedings, lectures, and public oral presentations. The psychologists' code also makes reference to the professional's continued responsibility to make *reasonable* efforts to insure that statements made on one's behalf are ethical. In other words, the psychologist cannot simply deny responsibility for misleading statements made in a promoter's announcement of a workshop simply because he or she did not write it. Another interesting aspect of the psychologists' code of ethics is that it no longer (as it did in the past) underscores psychologists' obligation to be accurate and honest in their public statements. Rather, as a result of a review by the Federal Trade Commission which took an interest in the ethics code as a potential restraint-of-trade tool, psychologists must "not make public statements that are false, deceptive, misleading, or fraudulent" (American Psychological Association, 1992, §3.03a). This is a somewhat more limited standard but still does convey the sense that one must not knowingly mislead or deceive the audience for one's statements.

Testimonials are an interesting problem. In some forms of mental health service, testimonials are an accepted business practice (e.g., organizational consulting, personal growth workshops). The difficulty with soliciting psychotherapy clients or ex-clients for testimonial purposes is that this may, on the one hand, be misleading to audiences (it is a distorted sample of consumers) and, on the other hand, may exploit the dependency and trust of the client. Thus, the psychologists' code specifies that psychologists "do not solicit testimonials from current psychotherapy clients or patients or other persons who because of their particular circumstances are vulnerable to undue influence" (American Psychological Association, 1992, §3.05).

With regard to testimonials, the social workers' code of ethics suggests indirectly that this is a problem. Principle D2 (NASW, 1993) specifies that "The social worker should not exploit professional relationships for personal gain" (§D.2.). Similarly, Principle F.2. states that "The social worker should not exploit relationships with clients for personal advantage" (§F.2.). With regard to other public statements, "the social worker should make no misrepresentation in advertising as to qualifications, competence, or results to be achieved" (§V.M.4.).

With regard to public statements, the marriage and family therapist "exercises special care" in making public statements (AAMFT, 1991, §3.8). He or she also must take reasonable precautions to insure his or her published materials are promoted accurately and factually (AAMFT, 1991). The AAMFT code has an entire section on advertising; in essence, it mandates honesty and accuracy. Interestingly, this can only be inferred from the language of the code. In keeping with current legal restrictions, the AAMFT code defines a false, fraudulent, misleading, or deceptive statement as one which contains a material misrepresentation of fact, fails to state any material fact necessary to make the statement, in light of all circumstances, not misleading, or is intended to or is likely to create an unjustified expectation.

The AAMFT code also underscores the professional's obligation to correct wherever possible misleading or inaccurate information or representations made about him or her.

Only the psychiatrists' code of ethics deals directly with the presentation of patients or former patients to a public gathering or the news media. This is considered ethical if the patient is fully informed of the consequences and consents in writing (American Psychiatric Association, 1993, p. 7).

Interestingly, the psychiatrists' code includes public statements under the section devoted to physicians' responsibility to participate in activities contributing to an improved community. This seems correct but interesting nonetheless. Psychiatrists are specifically prohibited from rendering opinions about individuals in the public eye unless the physician has actually examined that person and has been granted permission to release a statement.

An additional issue raised by self-promotional public statements is that of responsibility. It is not uncommon for third parties to edit or produce statements about a practitioner. Despite this fact, it is the practitioner's responsibility to insure that statements are accurate and not misleading. Thus to claim that the book publisher distorted one's qualifications in composing the advertising for a book is to ignore the ethical mandate that one is responsible for one's professional activities. In general, it is wise to obtain "review and revision rights" from third parties who are publishing such material. In addition, if there is doubt about the accuracy of one's statements, peer review or ethics committee consultation should be sought. An issue of recent vintage is the accuracy of statements made about the practitioner by managed care networks that include him or her on their panels (Stromberg, 1992).

PUBLIC STATEMENTS
ABOUT GENERAL TOPICS

Consider the following example. A professional practitioner and researcher is asked to appear on a local television show to discuss her research on sex role differences. Although the results of her research are interesting, they are fairly specific and have limited generalizability. The interviewer, however, repeatedly asks such questions as, "Yes, but don't you think men today are unable to handle women's changing roles?" or "Why are men so out of touch with their feelings?" The research that was conducted did not bear on these questions.

Not uncommonly, practitioners are asked to provide information to the public about general topics. These requests may take the form of interviews in print or on the air (via television or radio) and frequently focus on some topic agreed upon in advance. Here the issues are related to those noted before but are somewhat broader. That is, the practitioner must be scrupulously honest in what he or she says. It is all too easy, under pressure, to say something clever or provocative and overstep the bounds of fact or the bounds of one's competence. It is humbling (but ethically obligatory) to point out that one is not an expert on a topic that is in fact beyond one's competence. Inevitably, questioners or interviewers will touch on these topics and, in the interest of entertaining or stimulating their audience, may insist on an answer. It is hard to convey in written form the seductive pressures induced by an insistent interviewer under bright lights with television cameras rolling. Mental health professionals often want to please and will continue to speak when they should have stopped. Nonetheless these pressures must be resisted by the ethically responsible practitioner. Preparation for such situations is better than reaction, and "rehearsals" with trusted peers may be effective.

PUBLIC STATEMENTS
ABOUT SPECIFIC PROBLEMS

It is possible that when providing information about general topics, the practitioner can qualify his or her answers by noting that these are general issues that may not apply to all persons. Increasingly, however, practitioners are being asked to participate in live electronic media events which expose them to questions by specific persons about specific problems. These include phone-in talk shows, self-help shows, advice columns, and even computer bulletin-board-type interactive question-and-answer formats. Such circumstances are quite risky for the ethically responsible practitioner. A fundamental problem concerns divided loyalties, because the practitioner is being asked to use the caller's problem as a means of entertainment for the other members of the audience. At the same time, the practitioner has an ethical obligation to help the caller. Providing help to a particular caller may be misleading to listeners who do not share the specifics of the person's circumstances. For example, a caller who requests help with marital problems may seem to have circumstances similar to those of another listener with marital problems, but there may in fact be major differences. One may be married to a sadistic psychopath while the other may be married to an individual who simply lacks communication skills. It is important that the practitioner handle his or her responses in a way that misleads neither person.

In addition, as in the cases noted previously, the pressures to overstep the boundaries of one's competence are quite substantial. This is not simply a result of the demand characteristics of the television or radio studio; it may also be a result of the caller's providing limited information and time for extensive questioning being unavailable. It is usually not possible in such circumstances to take refuge in denials of responsibility; the fact that the producers of the show do not allow the practitioner enough time to adequately assess the caller's circumstances is not a valid defense against charges that the practitioner who gives a hasty and inadequate response is acting irresponsibly and unethically.

It is worthy of note that the American Psychological Association now includes a division of media psychology. There are peer support groups, consultation resources, and evolving standards in this area that would be of considerable help to the practitioner who is considering entering the public domain in such a fashion. Keith-Spiegel and Koocher (1985) cite additional developments in this area as well.

It is also worthy of note that there are ethical principles that might well be served by public media appearances. For example, media input might allow those too inhibited or constrained to seek professional help directly to receive at least some beneficial professional opinion. The preventive aspects of media psychology may also make a contribution to the quality of life. Thus the ethically responsible practitioner should not automatically refuse invitations for media appearances as too ethically troublesome. If the opportunity to make an impact through this avenue is appealing, careful preparation and self-discipline will be important.

GUIDELINES

1. *It is not possible to avoid responsibility for public statements.* For example, the responsible professional cannot take refuge in the fact that journalists might misquote him or her or misattribute the facts. Instead, the responsible professional insists on the opportunity to review, revise, or edit public statements if at all possible. Similarly, responsibility in broadcast media cannot be avoided by claiming that one was subjected to irresistible pressure to answer inappropriate questions. Instead, the responsible professional negotiates beforehand to insure his or her ability to refuse to answer inappropriate questions. This may also include insuring that a time delay is installed on the telephone used in call-in shows, so that one has a chance to screen calls. A further implication of this guideline is that not only must you have rights of review for statements made in your name or with your name attached, but also you should take steps to rectify whatever damage might be produced after a mis-statement has occurred. This may involve publishing retractions, amendments, follow-up TV shows, follow-up telephone calls to troubled callers, and so on.

2. *Don't overstep the boundaries of competence.* This means that practitioners must know what the boundaries of their competence *are*. It also means that practitioners must become skillful, perhaps by rehearsal, at reminding interviewers, callers, producers, and so on that their competence is not boundless.

3. *Be aware of potential conflicts of interest.* This includes reminding producers, publishers, interviewers, and so on of one's obligations to clients and potential clients as well as to the "host" of the particular medium in which one appears.

4. *Don't exploit callers.* This means that even though people naïvely ask for advice about apparently silly or inconse-

quential troubles, the practitioner must resist the temptation to exploit or mock them in a subtle way.

5. *Don't be afraid to seek consultation.* With the increasing body of knowledge accumulating in the area of media psychology, it is crucial to use this accumulated experience in preparing for media appearances.

Chapter 13

Psychological Testing
and Assessment Devices

A tremendous range of instruments purporting to measure mental status, neuropsychological functioning, personality makeup, marital communication, intellectual capacity, vocational interests, moral development, and the like is available to the modern mental health practitioner. Although psychological tests can be extremely useful in resolving diagnostic questions and developing effective treatment strategies, they can also be misused. Further, although testing is typically considered the domain of psychologists because of their expertise with various psychological tests, all mental health practitioners are likely to have to deal with the dilemmas that the proliferation of tests present. Whether psychologist or not, clinicians may have questions about their clients that some form of testing would answer; they may receive test results on their clients from other clinicians or clinics; or they may be asked by clients to arrange for an evaluation to answer specific questions. For this reason, ethical issues related to testing are relevant to all practitioners, not just to psychologists. However, the unique role of psychologists with regard to testing makes certain ethical issues particularly relevant to them. To deal with these separate issues, this chapter will be divided into two sections. The first will cover those aspects of testing that are relevant to all practitioners, and the second will highlight those issues specifically of concern to psychologists (as well as to other disciplines with psychological testing within their defined scope of practice).

GENERAL ISSUES IN TESTING

Because, as mentioned, all clinicians are likely to be involved with assessment in some form, there are certain ethical considerations that must be kept in mind. Those to be discussed here include practicing within one's area of expertise, sharing assessment information with clients in appropriate ways, and computerized assessment.

PRACTICING WITHIN ONE'S AREA OF EXPERTISE

With testing, as with any other area of clinical practice, it is important that practitioners know the "boundaries" of their competence. Several factors make assessment especially fertile ground for *boundary crossing*: first is the accessibility of testing material. Vendors of psychological tests are required in principle to restrict access to test materials to those with the appropriate credentials, but in practice it is extremely difficult to limit access to tests despite the sincere efforts of many vendors to do so. Thus clinicians often can purchase tests that they are not qualified to administer or interpret. Because of this, the burden is on each practitioner to be aware of the standards of training and knowledge required to administer a particular test.

A second important issue is that tests often seem easier to interpret than they really are. Frequently, interpretive reports of scale scores allow practitioners to think that they understand what a test means when in actuality they do not. The Minnesota Multiphasic Personality Inventory (MMPI; Hathaway & McKinley, 1943) and its revision (MMPI-2; Hathaway & McKinley, 1989) may be the most visible examples of this sort of problem. Practitioners who know the names of the various scales, as well as the mean and standard deviation of the scales, may feel qualified to interpret the test. However, such individuals are often blissfully unaware of several intricacies of the tests, including the facts that scale names and what they actually measure are often highly divergent, that the patterns or profiles of elevations are typically much more significant than individual scale elevations, that the configuration of the validity scales is of great importance, and so on. Further, the circumstances under which the test was administered and the emotional and motivational state of the test taker can greatly influence results. Although the MMPI is a clear-cut example of such problems, it is by no means the only example, and difficulties encountered by patients wrongly diagnosed in this fashion, or individuals made anxious or given inappropriate treatment based on incorrectly interpreted or scored tests are among the possible outcomes.

Illustrative of how the MMPI may be misinterpreted by untrained users is the case of the nurse who looked over a client's MMPI profile and commented on how passive-dependent the client was. When asked how she had come to this conclusion, she replied, "Look how high his Pd score is" (Pd is actually the abbreviation for "Psychopathic deviate," which in itself is a somewhat misleading label for the constellation of traits measured in this scale). As a further illustration, a social worker speculated that, based on MMPI results, it appeared that one of his clients was homosexual, until it was pointed out to him that he was using a female profile sheet (MMPI-2 profiles are slotted on different forms for males and females), thus causing the Mf (Masculinity-Femininity) Scale to be inaccurate. This example highlights two facts which a competent administrator of the test should know - first, the fact that male and female profile forms exist, and second, the relationship (or lack thereof) between Mf scores and homosexuality.

The solutions to these problems are largely ones of individual responsibility, of practitioners bearing the responsibility to know the limits of their competence. Responsible clinicians should know the acceptable scope of practice of their own discipline as codified in the ethical principles of that discipline, in published standards, and in relevant licensing laws. If practitioners are confronted by assessment questions with which they are not qualified to deal, referral to or consultation with an appropriately qualified colleague is in order.

SHARING ASSESSMENT
RESULTS WITH CLIENTS

Practitioners may encounter situations in which they are requested to share assessment results with clients, even if they themselves did not perform the assessment. For instance, there may be cases in which the client was referred to another professional for testing, but no feedback was given by the evaluator. Rather, the treating therapist has the responsibility to inform the client of the results. In presenting assessment information, there is a wide range of attitudes regarding what is appropriate (Berndt, 1983). Some clinicians believe that honesty is the ruling principle, and as a consequence share all results with the client without "editing." Other therapists opt for a more paternalistic stance, contending that the client has no need to know certain information and that it is up to the professional to decide what results are beneficial to share with the client.

From an ethical perspective, it may be useful to think of the decision regarding what assessment information to share as being based on the process of balancing informed consent (embodied in the principle of autonomy) with the clinician's responsibility to protect client welfare (embodied in the principle of beneficence). The practical implication of this perspective is that in most cases, the client has a right to know everything that results indicate about him or her unless the information would prove harmful in some way (and perhaps even then in certain limited cases). For instance, the clinician may, in certain circumstances, consider it countertherapeutic for a client to know that he or she has a low IQ score or has a tendency toward thought disorder. The therapist may then be justified in withholding certain assessment results or in presenting the information in a simplified, digestible form. It would, of course, be consistent with the obligation to promote client welfare to present assessment results in a therapeutic, or at least not countertherapeutic, manner. For instance, the comments, "You seem to have difficulty maintaining stable relationships" and "You have borderline personality tendencies" may convey the same concept, but one is probably less harmful (as well as more clinically sound) than the other.

Before sharing assessment information with the client, it is important to be sure that the circumstances of assessment are such that the clinician can ethically do so. For instance, if there is confusion regarding who the client is, as discussed in Chapter 8, then the practitioner should be certain that he or she is justified in sharing assessment information with the client. A clinician working in a correctional or other institutional setting, for example, does not necessarily have the same freedom in sharing assessment information with the client as does a clinician in a private practice setting. In the institution, assessment information usually "belongs" to the institution rather than to the individual.

To summarize, when a practitioner is asked to share testing information with a client, the following questions should be considered:

1. Does the practitioner have the right to divulge the information, or does the information "belong" to someone else?
2. Will knowledge of the information be harmful to the client?
3. Are the complete testing results relevant, or should only parts of the information be shared?
4. Is it necessary to "translate" or revise the wording of the report to make the information understandable or useful to the client?

COMPUTERIZED ASSESSMENT

The recent dramatic increase in the availability of computerized test administration, scoring, and interpretation services has increased the amount of assessment information available to clinicians. However, a number of ethical problems and concerns have accompanied this development (Matarazzo, 1986; Ryabik, Olson, & Kleim, 1984). Virtually every practitioner - psychologist or not - may be able to buy a computer disk that generates testing interpretations which, at least in surface appearance, seem similar to the psychological evaluations that a psychologist would provide.

Such computerized scoring and interpretation services have proliferated dramatically in recent years. As mentioned, many test vendors have tight restrictions on whom they will sell tests to, but once the test is sold to a qualified individual, it is up to that individual to maintain test security. We suspect that the extent to which this security is maintained varies dramatically among individuals, especially when tests are bought for use by large clinics or agencies.

Although it may seem that trying to impose limitations on such resources reflects nothing more than professional territoriality, there are some very practical reasons to follow guidelines in using computerized assessment and interpretation. Specifically, although the output of computer programs can look very impressive, this output is based on tests developed by and interpreted by individual human beings. The chosen tests must have demonstrated reliability and validity for use in a particular setting with a particular client. The test scoring and interpretation must be accurate, valid, and appropriate. In sum, testing programs are no better than the humans behind them, although they give the impression of being comparable to objective physical laboratory measurements in their precision and apparent completeness. Using such reports without awareness of the facts can lead to difficulty as easily as can misuse of the test itself.

Relatedly, it is important to note that when psychologists conduct psychological evaluations, they use more than one source of assessment information, and the evaluation reflects the synthesis of these sources so as to compensate for the error introduced by single measures used alone. A computerized test interpretation may look similar to a psychological evaluation, but it will be based on only one instrument and will likely be much less accurate (Groth-Marnat, 1984). Further, a psychologist who conducts a psychological evaluation will have face-to-face contact with the test taker and will be able to consider the specific characteristics of the individual and the context in which the test is administered; this is not the case with computerized testing.

Section 2.08c of the *Ethical Principles of Psychologists and Code of Conduct* (American Psychological Association, 1992) covers the issue of test scoring and interpretation services. Included in this section is the statement, "Psychologists retain appropriate responsibility for the appropriate application, interpretation, and use of assessment instruments, whether they score and interpret such tests themselves or use automated or other services" (§2.08c). Beyond these ethical standards, the American Psychological Association (1986) and the American Association of State Psychology Boards (1985) have developed guidelines for computer-based assessment and interpretation that should be read by anyone using such resources. Among other things, these guidelines specify that practitioners should only purchase and use computerized assessment programs that have demonstrated reliability and validity in the computerized form, that computerized assessments should only be conducted under circumstances similar to the ones in which they were validated, that the practitioner should use computer-generated reports only in the context of professional judgment and direct contact with the test taker, and that material taken from computer-generated interpretations should be identified as such.

One illustration of the harm that can come from uncontrolled computerized assessment occurred when a university student obtained an MMPI administration scoring and interpretation disk. After she had completed the test, the computer scored it and began printing an interpretation of her scores. As she watched, the computer printed page after page of highly pejorative statements about her functioning, including how she would likely destroy relationships and hurt her friends. Naturally this young woman was extremely upset as a result. Without strong controls over computerized assessment materials, similar unfortunate circumstances could easily proliferate.

ISSUES OF SPECIFIC
RELEVANCE TO PSYCHOLOGISTS

As noted, Standard 2 of the *Ethical Principles of Psychologists and Code of Conduct* (American Psychological Association, 1992) is devoted to ethical issues related to assessment techniques. In addition, the American Psychological Association, in cooperation with the American Educational Research Association and the

National Council on Measurement in Education, has published *Standards for Educational and Psychological Testing* (American Educational Research Association et al., 1985).   The material presented here should not be substituted for these two documents, but rather should be used as a summary of relevant concepts.

Beyond the expectations described in the previous sections of this chapter, the role of the psychologist implies other responsibilities in the process of assessment.   What follows is a summary listing of some of the ethical considerations a psychologist should keep in mind.   The considerations will be listed as a series of questions that the psychologist should ask himself or herself. Although some issues not covered below could be generated, our belief is that dealing satisfactorily with the questions below would provide a large measure of confidence in the ethical appropriateness of testing practices.

TEST SELECTION, ADMINISTRATION, AND SCORING

1. Do the tests selected have acceptable psychometric properties based on current information?
2. Are the selected tests appropriate for the intended use?
3. Are the selected tests appropriate for the intended population?
4. Is the examiner competent and qualified to administer and interpret the selected tests?

WELFARE OF THE TEST TAKER

1. Has the test taker given informed consent regarding testing procedures and use of results?
2. Is the testing environment conducive to test taking and free of distractions?

SHARING OF TEST RESULTS

1. Has an acceptable release of information been signed, or is there some reason that such a release is unnecessary?

2. Can the person(s) receiving results be trusted to use them responsibly and sensitively? What security is there to prevent further release of the information?
3. Is more information being released than is necessary?
4. Is care being taken to avoid inappropriate labeling of the test taker?
5. Will results be conveyed to the test taker (either by the psychologist who administered the testing or by someone else) in a responsible, sensitive manner? If there are negative emotional consequences, is there a system for dealing with them therapeutically?

SAFEGUARDING TESTING MATERIALS AND RESULTS

1. Are test materials secured to prevent access and use by unqualified individuals?
2. Are test results stored in such a way as to protect the test taker's rights of confidentiality? For instance, if results are in a computer file, is there adequate security?
3. Is there a system for eliminating obsolete test results from charts or files?

CONCLUDING COMMENTS

Tests and testing results can be an important source of clinical information and a potent source of conflict as well. Wright (1981) noted that disputes over psychological testing were the second most frequent causes of malpractice actions (after disputes regarding fees). Although this is, strictly speaking, primarily a psychologist's problem, other professionals should be aware that their use of tests and test results is both an opportunity and a risk. Increasingly, professionals must realize that they cannot afford to ignore the ever-more-sophisticated arsenal of tests available to them. At the same time, professionals have a clear obligation to use tests in a careful, appropriate manner.

Chapter 14

Forensic Mental Health: Practitioners in the Courtroom

It seems unlikely that any mental health practitioner could be in practice for very long without having some contact with the justice system. Often this experience comes through involvement in courtroom proceedings. For some, the court experience is eagerly anticipated and sought out. For others, the receipt of a subpoena or a call from an attorney engenders panic. We consider it important for mental health practitioners, even those who do not specialize in forensic work, to understand some of the issues, temptations, and pitfalls encountered in interfacing with the court system, so that they may be ready for their "day in court."

The seductive power of the courtroom, and the subtle gratification of being an expert, can sometimes blind the mental health professional to the need for particular skills and particular frames of mind necessary to both serve the court system and "do justice" to the complexity and integrity of the psychological issues at stake.

Partly in response to this state of affairs, there is increasing interest in the field regarding the tactics and strategies of "expert witnessing" (e.g., Brodsky, 1991; Shapiro, 1990). Much of this advice focuses on the mechanics of testifying; there is at least a modicum of attention paid to the notion of preparing properly, recognizing the boundaries of competence, and so forth. Judging by the sorts of complaints that reach ethics committees and licensing boards, however, more professional attention needs to be addressed to the issues of competence and quality in psychological courtroom work.

Of course, most, if not all, of the other concepts discussed in this book have applications to the legal setting. These would include confidentiality and privilege, competence, dual relationships, loyalty conflicts, and so on. However, given the unique nature of the court system and the mental health practitioner's role within it, it seems appropriate to devote a chapter specifically to court issues and their ethical implications.

Much work has been done discussing the role of the forensic mental health professional and the ethical considerations implicit in this role (e.g., Applebaum, 1990; Golding, 1990; Melton et al., 1987). It should be made clear that the field of forensics is a fairly well-developed subspecialty, at least in psychology and psychiatry. Thus, board certification is available in both forensic psychology and forensic psychiatry, there are training programs in these areas, and so forth. There are also abundant sets of professional guidelines for the forensic psychologist (e.g., Division of Psychology and Law, 1991). The present discussion should not substitute for detailed study if one wishes to specialize in forensic mental health work; nevertheless, in the recognition that nonspecialist clinicians may be called upon to provide testimony or otherwise make contact with the legal system, we offer some introductory concepts. Additional sources should be consulted and further training should be obtained if one desires to pursue this further. The present chapter is intended as an overview of the ethical considerations specifically relevant to dealing with the courts and is intended for those practitioners not specializing in courtroom work. For clarity, we will deal separately with situations where one is in court with one's client and when one is dealing with nonclients. These issues are relevant to questions of competence, as discussed in Chapter 3. The key ethical dimension here is whether one is serving one's clients by offering forensic mental health services when one is not well acquainted with the legal arena.

Competence in this arena, at least in part, represents the competence to balance the competing interests of scientific objectivity and advocacy, to speak to a largely lay audience without trivializing or overgeneralizing findings, to maintain the ethical obligations (beneficence, autonomy, nonmaleficence), and to understand and implement the specifics of one's ethical code.

TESTIFYING ABOUT ONE'S CLIENT

Practitioners may be called to testify in court either by their client or by the opposing side. Which side initiates the request (or order) is critically important in determining what the practitioner does. Each of these contexts will be discussed in turn.

GIVING TESTIMONY
REQUESTED BY THE CLIENT

If the request comes from the client himself or herself, then worries about breaching privilege are minimal, because privilege is the client's to waive. However, for self-protection, a signed release of information from the client would be advisable. The implications of testifying should be discussed with the client in advance, as well. For example, could cross-examination take you beyond the area in which the client wished you to testify? If the privilege is waived by requesting your testimony, does this waive it *entirely*?

In order to minimize confusion or misunderstanding, if the client has initially sought treatment because it was court-ordered or under other circumstances which would likely lead to courtroom involvement, these and related issues should be discussed and resolved at the beginning of treatment, and the therapist's role clarified at the outset.

Clients should be aware that they cannot restrict you to testifying only about the good things that they do and that your testimony will be subject to cross-examination. Although you can say that your testimony will be limited only to relevant information, relevance is a legal determination once you are in court. If the client's attorney does not object to a question raised in cross-examination, or the judge orders you to answer a question over the attorney's objections, then you have to do so, even if you and the client consider it irrelevant.

As mentioned in the chapter on confidentiality, there is the troubling situation in which a therapist has seen more than one family member, for instance in marriage or family counseling. If some individuals are willing to waive privilege and some not, then the therapist can testify only about those individuals who have given permission. Trying to extract information only about certain individuals seen in a system context can be very tricky. Resolving these problems and deciding what can and cannot be said should be a matter negotiated among the therapist, the parties involved, and their counsel, as well as possibly the judge.

GIVING TESTIMONY REQUESTED BY THE OPPOSING SIDE

If one's client is involved in a legal proceeding and the opposing side seeks the testimony, then the first issue for the practitioner to consider relates to whether privilege can be breached. As mentioned previously (see Chapter 4), the mere receipt of a subpoena does not allow you to breach privilege. Practitioners should seek their own legal advice upon receiving a subpoena as well as consulting with the client and the client's attorney. In some cases, the client may freely waive privilege; the clinician's ethical responsibility, as before, is to insure that this is done with full awareness of the potential consequences. In other cases, the nature of the judicial proceedings may motivate the court to breach the client's privilege or may represent an automatic waiver of privilege. Examples of such situations would include suspected child abuse or a situation in which the client has entered his or her own mental state into the judicial proceedings. However, even if it seems obvious to you that the situation involves an implicit waiver of privilege, this should still be legally determined. That is, you would be wise always to claim privilege and then be ordered by the court to breach it.

Regardless of how the practitioner finds himself or herself in court, once there, and once the practitioner's testimony is allowed, other ethical questions are likely to occur. For one thing, dual relationship issues will probably emerge. However the practitioner characterizes his or her relationship with the client in the treatment setting (e.g., as a doctor whose purpose is to heal; as a consultant in living), courtroom testimony raises other roles for the practitioner: as an advocate, as an objective and detached evaluator, or possibly even as an antagonist. This can lead to a number of potential ethical violations, including betrayal or abandonment of the client (or at least the perception thereof).

Further, the adversarial nature of the courtroom procedure complicates the practitioner's role, in that there is considerable demand to present only that information that furthers one side or the other (Shapiro, 1992). Such a practice would be unethical, because biased information would be presented under the guise of scientific objectivity and detachment.

The competent expert should also know what he or she has *not* done, as well as what he or she has done (Shapiro, 1990). This question is likely to be brought out by opposing counsel in any case, because the attempt to discredit the expert witness will involve the inadequacy of the assessment or evaluation (Shapiro, 1990, notes, ". . . there is a constant temptation in forensic work to go beyond the limits of one's competence and to render opinions in areas in which either the psychologist has no particular training or the state of knowledge is so meager that opinions should not be rendered" [p. 746]).

Based on the preceding issues, we recommend some steps that a practitioner should take in providing court testimony about a client. The first is a restatement of something emphasized throughout this book - that it is wise to anticipate the potential for court involvement and to plan accordingly. Second, be clear as to your role vis-à-vis the court - to yourself, to your client, and to the court itself. If you have been a therapist to an individual, it must be clear to everyone involved that you should not be seen as an unbiased evaluator. Third, we consider it inappropriate from an ethical perspective to withhold information from the court. However, this statement must be clarified. Given the way court testimony works, you will be asked to respond to specific questions, and it is ethically appropriate to answer these questions honestly, even if your answers hurt your client. However, you are under no obligation to share information that is not sought. It is up to each attorney to elicit from you the information he or she wants, and, even if you consider information germane, it is not appropriate for you to volunteer it.

COURTROOM ROLES
WITH NONCLIENTS

There are many roles a clinician can play in the courtroom in addition to the one mentioned previously. Examples can include conducting child custody evaluations, testimony as an expert witness about areas in which one has particular expertise, and conducting specialized evaluations for the court (e.g., competency, diminished capacity, guilty but mentally ill).

Garb (1991) in a useful discussion of the expert witness's task, notes that an expert witness should be able to help a judge or jury make more accurate judgments. If an expert witness cannot make more valid judgments than a judge or jury, then it is unlikely that the expert will be able to help a judge or jury improve the accuracy of their judgments (Garb, 1991, p. 452).

As mentioned, if one is considering doing a lot of courtroom work or doing work of a highly technical nature, then this should be considered specialty work and the standards of training and competence should be commensurate. Custody evaluations and the specialized types of evaluations noted previously are examples. However, as a function of their area of specialization, practitioners without specific forensic training may be called upon to testify as expert witnesses. Following are listed some of the common ethical considerations and pitfalls in this role.

SPECIAL PREROGATIVES
OF THE EXPERT WITNESS

Once an individual is qualified by the court as an expert witness, he or she is given a status not accorded nonexpert witnesses (Golding, 1990). Specifically, an expert witness can testify as to opinions and inferences. If a nonexpert witness presents such inferences and speculations, they are disqualified. With this authority comes a greater ethical responsibility, in that we must be sensitive to the special influence conferred by the simple fact of being an expert witness. The courtroom setting is very seductive and can provide fertile ground for an expert witness to "expound" on his or her opinions and go beyond what can be supported (Keith-Spiegel & Koocher, 1985). This temptation should, of course, be avoided.

THE EXPERT WITNESS ROLE

Practitioners not accustomed to courtroom work may assume a role different from the one that is appropriate. As Weissman (1991) has stated, the expert witness is not an advocate (the attorney's role) nor the trier of fact (the judge's role). One implication of this statement is that, although the expert witness can provide information, it is up to the judge to make the final decision.

Another implication of the preceding statement is that an expert witness is obligated to present information in as objective and detached a manner as possible. There are a number of reasons that an expert witness can feel considerable pressure to distort or slant the data, present only arguments that support one side, or go beyond what can competently be asserted. First, there may be the feeling that if one gives testimony supportive of the side that hired him or her, there will be more such business in the future (the "hired gun"). Second, attorneys can be quite persuasive and seductive in eliciting the desired information and can "turn the expert witness's head" in very subtle ways. Although this may be seen as cause for cynicism and "attorney bashing," it must be remembered that the basis of our legal system is that the attorney is an advocate for the client and must present the best case possible. Indeed the attorney is ethically obligated to advocate as best he or she can for his or her client's cause. Is the psychologist in court more like the attorney? It is interesting to note that faith in the legal adversarial system requires that lawyers become aggressive, competitive, and technically oriented. It is nowhere near as clear what might be the appropriate stance for psychologists.

Another pressure may be especially strong for mental health professionals and is discussed separately in the next section.

CONFLICTS OF ETHICAL PRINCIPLES

Many practitioners are used to a clinical setting, in which principles of beneficence and nonmaleficence are paramount. The testimony of an expert witness can be extremely damaging to someone involved in the court proceedings (Applebaum, 1990). To distort the truth or withhold information, even in the service of promoting good or avoiding harm, would be considered unethical. Because of this, Applebaum (1990) has contended that ethical principles in the courtroom should be looked at as different from those in clinical settings.

DIFFERENCES BETWEEN LEGAL
AND MENTAL HEALTH CONCEPTS

One of the important considerations in doing courtroom work relates to the differences between legal and mental health concepts, and it is important for the practitioner to be aware of these differences (Keith-Spiegel & Koocher, 1985). The ethical principle involved here is one of competence. That is, the expert witness should have an understanding of how mental health terms translate into legal terms, as relevant to the matter at hand. For instance, it is important to be able to differentiate mental illness as defined by statute from what one's own clinical definition of mental illness is (e.g., as synonymous with psychosis).

He or she will also have the judgment to know what is missing, and in which areas his or her conclusions need to be tempered, qualified, or limited. Garb (1991) notes, "even when mental health professionals cannot make moderately accurate predictions they can still assist judges and juries. For example, they can describe the appropriate empirical research and simply conclude that the prediction task is difficult or they may be able to help select appropriate statistical decision rules" (p. 453).

Shapiro (1990) also notes that expert witnesses must remain objective and impartial regardless of which side retains his or her services. In practice this seems rather difficult to achieve, in that one's income derives from one side or the other. Nonetheless, the standard to which one should aspire is that one's opinion is based on the data and is not contaminated by one's association with plaintiff or defendant. Clearly the opposing side will try to establish that this is not the case.

Another problem is that forensic psychological activities have yet to be as carefully assessed for their potential to do harm. Indeed, in a recent ethics complaint, the psychologist defended himself by noting that the court failed to follow his recommendations (which were based on inadequate assessment) and therefore no harm came to the complainant. This is a spurious defense, but it rests on a common belief of less than competent psychologists; that is, the belief that the adversarial legal system can "protect itself" and screen out incompetent psychologists through courtroom procedures, rules of evidence, expert qualifying processes, and the like. Yet the ethical perspective on professional competence leads us to consider psychologists' own interests, whether or not the legal system has safeguards, in practicing at the highest level of competence and certainly to practice with the aim of minimizing potential harm (nonmaleficence; Beauchamp & Childress, 1979).

PROBLEMS

1. *Lack of fidelity.* This is exemplified by the expert witness who changes his position between the time of agreeing with the attorney to testify and actually appearing in court. Another example might be the therapist who works with a couple on resolving their marital stresses and appears in court on behalf of only one member of the couple to argue for custody.
2. *Lack of prudence.* This difficulty might be illustrated by the case of a psychologist who uses obsolete test results.
3. *Lack of discretion.* This might be illustrated by the psychologist who casually diagnoses the member of a couple whom she has not seen in treatment as "obviously a borderline."
4. *Lack of integrity.* This might be illustrated by the expert witness who confidently reconstructs a conversation held in therapy 15 years earlier without benefit of notes.

5. *Lack of humility.* This might be illustrated by the expert witness who claims on the witness stand he can invariably detect schizophrenia.

The abundance of ethics complaints to ethics committees and licensing boards about the actions of psychologists in the court-room suggests that the demanding characteristics of the forensic arena exert considerable pressure on even highly trained psychologists to abandon the standards of excellence they might espouse in calmer environments. The pressures of being on the witness stand and the seductions of extravagantly compensated evaluations and testimony can lead to enormous temptations to be a "hired gun" for the side that obtains one's services.

Chapter 15

Clinical Research
in Real-Life Practice

Why is there a chapter (albeit a short chapter) on clinical research in an ethics primer for practitioners? The fundamental reason is that the mental health professions distinguish themselves from spiritual, religious, or charismatic self-improvement techniques by virtue of the grounding of mental health practice in scientific evidence. Clinicians belong to a professional culture that is committed to creating and evolving an empirical foundation for its work. Thus, implicitly or explicitly, mental health practitioners must have a perspective on the linkage between ethical practice and their approach to research activities. In the mental health professions' codes of ethics, it is stated or implied that advancing the sciences contributing to improved mental health is an ethical obligation of the practitioner. Social workers (NASW, 1993), for instance, "take responsibility for identifying, developing, and fully utilizing knowledge for professional practice" (§V.O.). Psychologists "are concerned about and work to mitigate the causes of human suffering. When undertaking research, they strive to advance human welfare and the science of psychology" (American Psychological Association, 1992, Principle F). Physicians "shall continue to study, apply, and advance scientific knowledge" (American Psychiatric Association, 1992, §5). In the pursuit of these goals, even practitioners who do not themselves conduct empirical studies may be called upon to cooperate in others' clinical research activities. It is likely that even the solo independent practitioner will have opportunities to participate in clinical research at one or more points in a career. In addition to its service to the field of mental health in general, such participation can be personally and professionally rewarding to the practitioner. It is important that practitioners outside of the academic setting be involved in clinical research, because, in the absence of such involvement, it would be more likely that studies would be artificial and unrealistic. This chapter briefly reviews the pros and cons of participating in such research and highlights some of the dilemmas inherent in the major ethical issue, which is protecting the welfare of one's patients while advancing the scientific progress of one's discipline.

PRIMARY ETHICAL ISSUES

The practitioner's involvement in clinical research involves three major ethical issues: First, there is the consideration of wise investment of time. Practitioners must decide what sort of research is likely to be meaningful to themselves and their patients. Second, one must minimize dual relationships. Involvement in clinical research can present a loyalty conflict between responding to the needs of patients and responding to the requirements of the study. Third, involvement in clinical research highlights the ethical obligation to promote the well-being of one's patients and to provide them informed consent. For example, practitioners must carefully assess the protection of patient identities and the effectiveness of informed-consent procedures.

THE PRACTITIONER'S RESPONSIBILITY

Ethical practitioners must have the option to decline participation in clinical research if it appears that the investment of their time and their patients' time will not result in any meaningful benefits either to the patients or the field as a whole. This can be a difficult judgment to make, especially if one is not an expert in the proposed area of research. In such cases it is necessary to rely on the judgment of the principal investigator, although one cannot abandon responsibility for making this judgment in the final analysis. Second, one cannot remove one's patients' autonomy by enrolling them in a clinical study without their consent. The patients must be informed, especially if the study involves any changes in the treatment that they would ordinarily get. Third, the practitioner must insure that opportunities are available for detecting and remedying any negative effects which may result from the research involvement. For example, if some of the practitioner's patients are assigned to a waiting list or a "placebo control" group, the practitioner must reserve the option of providing some sort of treatment to these patients should their distress increase. The primary investigator should bear significant responsibility for the preceding concerns. However, a practitioner whose clients are involved in the research must also bear the responsibility for the maintenance of ethical conduct and procedures. He or she should avoid passive acquiescence to questionable practices, even in dealing with senior investigators with impressive research and academic credentials. An issue that is troublesome for many practitioners involves informing patients about their assignment to treatment versus control groups. If there is true random assignment, it is probably not in the interests of scientific validity to inform the patients of this, because those who are assigned to placebo or control groups may well withdraw from the study and thus bias the sample. On the other hand, patients have the right to know that random assignment will take place and must be willing to be assigned to the "other" condition. In general, the ethical researcher informs patients that assignment will take place, but may reserve the right not to inform the patients of the nature of the group to which they are assigned. A preferable resolution of this problem is to offer as the alternative treatment the best available treatment that is known for the patient's condition. If the study's principal investigator has not developed such an alternative treatment, it is the responsibility of the practitioner to attempt to educate the researcher.

GUIDELINES

Based on the preceding, the following guidelines may prove useful in deciding whether or not to participate in a research project.

1. *Is it a worthwhile project?* Will the project answer important, relevant questions? Will it answer questions of importance to practitioners or theorists?
2. *Has it passed through appropriate committees?* A
   university-sponsored project typically should have passed
   a human-subjects committee. If the practitioner is part of
   an agency, it might be appropriate for that agency to
   establish a committee to assure that the rights of subjects
   are protected. If there is no committee to protect subjects'
   rights, the clinician's responsibilities to do so are increased.
3. *Has the client given informed consent?* Although the
   purpose of the research may need to be withheld from the
   client, the client should be fully apprised of any information that may pertain to his or her decision to participate.
4. *Is there potential harm to the client? Do the benefits
   outweigh the harm?* This is obviously a very subjective
   decision, but the clinician should be able to be sure that
   there is minimal harm to the client and that the potential
   benefits outweigh any possible harm.
5. *Have appropriate safeguards been put into place for the
   client?* In the event of harm to the client, there should be
   remedial measures in place. The client should be free to
   withdraw at any time and should be aware of this freedom.

Chapter 16

Professional Renewal:
Avoiding "Practitioner Decay"

Mental health practice is both art and science. Although improvements in one's practice of the art of psychotherapy do not depend on keeping abreast of the literature, the scientific aspects of the mental health disciplines require that one be familiar with current knowledge (ironically known as "the state of the art"). The explosion of information available with regard to new methods of treatment, revised views of existing methods, and new findings concerning the sources and symptoms of psychopathology mean that mental health knowledge can be considered to have a relatively short "half-life." This concept is drawn from Dubin (1972), who estimated that the half-life of a doctoral degree in psychology (as a measure of competence) was 10 to 12 years. In other words, over a decade's time approximately half of one's original fund of knowledge becomes irrelevant or wrong. Similarly, Campbell and Stanley (1963) coined the term "instrument decay" to refer to the decrease over time in the quality of the instrument used to rate a phenomenon under study. Regardless of the analogy, the issue of professional obsolescence can be dealt with only by continuing efforts to stay abreast of developments in one's areas of practice. This is perhaps simply another way of underscoring the obligation to be competent, with the added perspective that "competence" is not a permanent state achieved when one obtains the necessary credentials, but rather a continuing process of improving and refining one's diagnostic and treatment skills. Described below are two general areas in which practitioner decay can be problematic: professional knowledge and professional judgment and balance. For each, some specific considerations and guidelines will be described.

PROFESSIONAL KNOWLEDGE

Practitioners have the obligation to stay abreast of current professional knowledge, and the ethical codes of psychiatry, social work, psychology, and marriage and family therapy all contain provisions to this effect. Although it may seem at times that the accepted body of professional knowledge in mental health fields grows at an imperceptibly slow rate and that we are perpetually rediscovering the wheel, when one compares the practice of psychotherapy now with practices of even a decade ago, there are numerous areas in which professional knowledge, techniques, and responsibilities have changed. Such areas as legal and ethical issues, the role of biological factors in behavioral problems, the role of distorted cognitions, advancements in diagnosis and assessment techniques, appropriate use of hypnosis, and treatment of sexual dysfunction are among the areas that have shown marked changes. Further, even more traditional techniques such as psychoanalysis and behavior modification have grown and evolved.

Although it is incumbent on the practitioner to stay current, the task of assessing whether one is actually up to date in a particular area of practice is often very difficult. A guideline that a practitioner may wish to use in this regard involves a practice attorneys sometimes employ in cross-examining an opposing expert witness. The witness is asked to identify the most significant works in a particular area of practice and to indicate which ones he or she has read. The practitioner who asks himself or herself these questions may be able to obtain an estimate of his or her level of knowledge in the area in question. It is our assumption that most practitioners earnestly desire to stay current in terms of professional developments and techniques. However, given the heavy service demands that most practitioners face and the emotional strain that practitioners encounter, it is understandable that the time and energy needed to stay current may be sacrificed.

When a clinician has spent a long day dealing with emotionally distressed individuals, the last thing he or she may want to do when arriving at home is to peruse journals. Further, when one considers the loss to a clinician's income that results from attending a 2- or 3-day seminar, it may be very tempting for many private practitioners to stay in the office and work instead.

The need to stay current has been recognized by many licensing authorities, and many licensing boards have established continuing-education requirements that must be met to maintain one's license or certification. In addition, in some states, it is necessary to provide evidence of continuing education to obtain malpractice insurance. Typically, however, such standards are minimal in scope and do little to focus attention on the content areas necessary to insure that a professional will stay current.

Whether or not one is in a situation in which continuing education is required, the professional must bear major responsibility for insuring exposure to advances in professional practice and changes in professional responsibilities. At a minimum, practitioners should subscribe to journals that are relevant to their practice and become familiar with the contents. It would be expected, in this regard, that practitioners will have the ability to assess the quality of the articles read, so that their practice is not guided by erroneous findings. The importance of this requirement is highlighted by the presence of such currently controversial topics as multiple personalities, ritual abuse, false memories, and so on. In areas such as these, there is a wide range of opinion, the debate can be extremely emotional, and the negative consequences to clients of misapplied or inaccurate knowledge can be significant. As a result, it is especially important for the practitioner to maintain knowledge of research methodology and be aware of potential sources of bias in the reporting of research. Because it is difficult to read articles in all relevant areas of practice, the practitioner may wish to have information presented in a digested or condensed version. "State of the art" lectures at national conventions are helpful, as are the opinions of senior colleagues regarding which professional journals have merit. Digesting or abstracting services have also become more widely available, including the following:

1. *Psychscan* (several available with specialty emphasis). This is an abbreviated literature search tool which provides citations and abstracts, as well as addresses to write to authors for reprints. It is available through the American Psychological Association (202-336-5600) and is offered at a reduced price for Association members. The address of the American Psychological Association is 750 First Street NE, Washington, DC 20002-4242.
2. *The Harvard Medical School Mental Health Letter.* This periodical is typically devoted to a theme (a particular disorder, or method of treatment) and also includes brief reports of current research. It is published by Harvard Medical School (800-829-5379). For ordering information, contact R. L. Polk & Company, 300 Atlantic Street, Stanford, CT 06901.
3. *Clinician's Research Digest.* Another source of brief article summaries from the psychological, psychiatric, and social work literature. Available from American Psychological Association, 750 First Street NE, Washington, DC 20002-4242. The phone number is 202-336-5600.

It must be remembered that many of these sources present information in a form that is difficult to evaluate methodologically, and there is a wide range of work cited, from the trivial and inaccurate to the profound and essential. It is important for the practitioner to assess the accuracy and relevance of the information presented. One option for helping the practitioner stay current involves the increased accessibility of computerized databases which contain references and abstracts of thousands of articles. These databases were once prohibitively expensive and available only to institutions, but they are now available to individuals with computers and modems and are reasonably inexpensive (if used conservatively). In a short period of time, a practitioner can enter key words and review relevant abstracts. Although these services take a little practice to use effectively, their benefit in keeping clinicians current can be significant. Three such services include:

1. *Knowledge Index* (an off-peak version of DIALOG literature retrieval and searching service; telephone: 800-334-
   2564). Charges a monthly fee. Can also be accessed
   through Compuserve (800-848-8990).
2. *BRS After Dark* (800-955-0906). Another abstract and
   citation retrieval service.
3. *Current Contents on Disk.* Extremely comprehensive set
   of abstracts from a wide range of social science journals,
   sent on disk monthly. User can construct personal search
   strategy and easily run it on each new disk. Offered by
   Institute for Scientific Information, 3501 Market Street,
   Philadelphia, PA 19104 (800-523-1850). Expensive.

As in the case of printed digests, practitioners bear added
responsibility to separate useful from trivial reports, because abstracting services are completely nonselective. As important as
having such resources available is maintaining the motivation to
use them on a regular basis. Individuals with good self-control
may have naturally good habits, or they may set up standards for
themselves (e.g., "I won't watch television until I have reviewed
10 abstracts"). The rest of us may have to compensate for our
lack of self-control by setting up a structure that requires us to
stay current. One good way to do so is to establish a relationship
with training institutions to provide ongoing contact with students.
While the practitioner is sharing his or her years of experience
with the student, the student is providing the practitioner with
information regarding current techniques, approaches, and so on.
Practitioners may also be able to make arrangements to teach
classes at a university, community college, or community school.
Although the financial rewards may be meager from such teaching, one's time is still compensated to a certain extent, and the
value to the practitioner is the enhancement of his or her knowledge. It is conventional wisdom that to learn best, one should
teach, and this is particularly true in mental health practice, because much of the work goes on without peer involvement. In
addition, the practitioner may find it useful to participate in journal clubs, case conferences, or similar professional activities.
Finally, the practitioner should maintain active involvement with

appropriate professional organizations and, if time allows, commit himself or herself to some function within the organization. Doing so gives the practitioner exposure to professional developments that is hard to obtain by interacting only with a journal or a computer terminal, and at the same time offers the opportunity to influence the development of one's own profession.

PROFESSIONAL JUDGMENT AND PROFESSIONAL BALANCE

There is a second component necessary for the practitioner to provide effective services to patients in addition to maintaining awareness of advances in the field. This second element involves the use of professional judgment in knowing when to use this knowledge or technique effectively. A key factor that may reduce the quality of professional judgment over time, and that needs to be considered in one's ongoing efforts to prevent professional decay, is burnout. A therapist who feels overwhelmed and stressed in dealing with clients may not only be uninterested in professional reading or attending professional meetings, but may also show higher levels of anger or blame toward clients, may attempt to terminate them prematurely, may not invest emotionally to the extent appropriate, or may, in some other unconscious way, act out the resentment that he or she feels at having the responsibility for patients' welfare. As Freudenberger (1982) and others have pointed out, mental health professionals are at high risk for "burning out" because of the large emotional commitment necessary and the frustratingly small visible gains from that investment. Mental health practitioners must operate in an environment of uncertain effects from their work and one in which they are frequently not appreciated for their helpfulness. A related process that can occur to practitioners over time involves a gradual decrease in attention they pay to other aspects of their own lives besides work and an inappropriate emphasis on therapeutic relationships to meet certain needs (discussed in Chapter 6). For instance, a therapist whose social life is restricted, for whatever reason, may seek to meet needs for affiliation through contact with clients, and his or her professional judgment may reflect this need

rather than the clients' best interests. All practitioners are suscep-
tible to decrements in professional judgment brought on by such
factors as burnout or "life imbalance," and all would be wise to
take steps to monitor and prevent such processes. A necessary
first step is open and sincere self-monitoring of one's motivations.
As alluded to previously in this book, humans are all capable of
significant levels of self-deception, and our status as therapists
does not make us any different. It is hoped, however, that therapists are more attuned to this risk than many other professionals
and are open to self-exploration as well as to the feedback of
others, even if such feedback is hard to take. In dealing with
decrements in professional judgment, practitioners are also wise to
continually monitor their lives to make sure that there is a balance
of work, social, and recreational activities. Although a practitioner's use of his or her own time is a personal matter, it has professional and ethical relevance when actions taken with clients are
affected.

In summary, therapists should include in responsible and
ethical practice efforts to take care of their own needs; it is not a
sign of selfishness if one does not devote every waking hour to
client care. In fact, we hope that the present discussion has suggested how such self-interest might make one a more effective
professional, as well as a happier one.

Appendices

Code of Ethics
American Association for
Marriage and Family Therapy (AAMFT)

**The Principles of Medical Ethics
With Annotations Especially
Applicable to Psychiatry**
American Psychiatric Association

**Ethical Principles of Psychologists
and Code of Conduct**
American Psychological Association

Code of Ethics
National Association of
Social Workers (NASW)

Appendix A

Code of Ethics
American Association for
Marriage and Family Therapy (AAMFT)*

1. RESPONSIBILITY TO CLIENTS

Marriage and family therapists advance the welfare of families and individuals. They respect the rights of those persons seeking their assistance, and make reasonable efforts to ensure that their services are used appropriately.

1.1 Marriage and family therapists do not discriminate against or refuse professional service to anyone on the basis of race, gender, religion, national origin, or sexual orientation.

1.2 Marriage and family therapists are aware of their influential position with respect to clients, and they avoid exploiting the trust and dependency of such persons. Therapists, therefore, make every effort to avoid dual relationships with clients that could impair professional judgment or increase the risk of exploitation. When a dual relationship cannot be avoided, therapists take appropriate professional precautions to ensure judgment is not impaired and no exploitation occurs. Examples of such dual relationships include, but are not limited to, business or close personal relationships with clients.

*Note: Reprinted from *AAMFT Code of Ethics*. This revised code was approved in August, 1991, copyright © 1991, American Association for Marriage and Family Therapy. Reprinted with permission. No additional copies may be made without obtaining permission from AAMFT.

Sexual intimacy with clients is prohibited. Sexual intimacy with former clients for two years following the termination of therapy is prohibited.

1.3   Marriage and family therapists do not use their professional relationships with clients to further their own interests.

1.4   Marriage and family therapists respect the right of clients to make decisions and help them to understand the consequences of these decisions. Therapists clearly advise a client that a decision on marital status is the responsibility of the client.

1.5   Marriage and family therapists continue therapeutic relationships only so long as it is reasonably clear that clients are benefiting from the relationship.

1.6   Marriage and family therapists assist persons in obtaining other therapeutic services if the therapist is unable or unwilling, for appropriate reasons, to provide professional help.

1.7   Marriage and family therapists do not abandon or neglect clients in treatment without making reasonable arrangements for the continuation of such treatment.

1.8   Marriage and family therapists obtain written informed consent from clients before videotaping, audiorecording, or permitting third party observation.

2.   CONFIDENTIALITY

Marriage and family therapists have unique confidentiality concerns because the client in a therapeutic relationship may be more than one person. Therapists respect and guard confidences of each individual client.

2.1   Marriage and family therapists may not disclose client confidences except: (a) as mandated by law; (b) to prevent a clear and immediate danger to a person or persons; (c) where the therapist is a defendant in a civil, criminal, or disciplinary action arising from the therapy (in which case client confidences may be disclosed only in the course of that action); or (d) if there is a waiver previously obtained in writing, and then such information may be revealed only in accordance with the terms of the waiver. In circumstances where more than one person in a family receives therapy, each such family member who is legally competent to execute a waiver must agree to the waiver required by subparagraph (d). Without such a waiver from each family member legally competent to execute a waiver, a therapist cannot disclose information received from any family member.

2.2   Marriage and family therapists use client and/or clinical materials in teaching, writing, and public presentations only if a written waiver has been obtained in accordance with Subprinciple 2.1(d), or when appropriate steps have been taken to protect client identity and confidentiality.

2.3   Marriage and family therapists store or dispose of client records in ways that maintain confidentiality.

3.   PROFESSIONAL COMPETENCE AND INTEGRITY

Marriage and family therapists maintain high standards of professional competence and integrity.

3.1   Marriage and family therapists are in violation of this Code and subject to termination of membership or other appropriate action if they: (a) are convicted of any felony; (b) are convicted of a misdemeanor related to their qualifications or functions; (c) engage in conduct which could lead to conviction of a felony, or a misdemeanor related to their qualifications or functions; (d) are expelled from or disciplined by other professional organizations; (e) have their licenses or certificates suspended or revoked or are otherwise disciplined by regulatory bodies; (f) are no longer competent to practice marriage and family therapy because they are impaired due to physical or mental causes or the abuse of alcohol or other substances; or (g) fail to cooperate with the Association at any point from the inception of an ethical complaint through the completion of all proceedings regarding that complaint.

3.2   Marriage and family therapists seek appropriate professional assistance for their personal problems or conflicts that may impair work performance or clinical judgment.

3.3   Marriage and family therapists, as teachers, supervisors, and researchers, are dedicated to high standards of scholarship and present accurate information.

3.4   Marriage and family therapists remain abreast of new developments in family therapy knowledge and practice through educational activities.

3.5   Marriage and family therapists do not engage in sexual or other harassment or exploitation of clients, students, trainees, supervisees, employees, colleagues, research subjects, or actual or potential witnesses or complainants in investigations and ethical proceedings.

3.6   Marriage and family therapists do not diagnose, treat, or advise on problems outside the recognized boundaries of their competence.

3.7   Marriage and family therapists make efforts to prevent the distortion or misuse of their clinical and research findings.

3.8   Marriage and family therapists, because of their ability to influence and alter the lives of others, exercise special care when making public their professional recommendations and opinions through testimony or other public statements.

4.   RESPONSIBILITY TO STUDENTS, EMPLOYEES, AND SUPERVISEES

Marriage and family therapists do not exploit the trust and dependency of students, employees, and supervisees.

4.1   Marriage and family therapists are aware of their influential position with respect to students, employees, and supervisees, and they avoid exploiting the trust and dependency of such persons. Therapists, therefore, make every effort to avoid dual relationships that could impair professional judgment or increase the risk of exploitation. When a dual relationship cannot be avoided, therapists take appropriate professional precautions to ensure judgment is not impaired and no exploitation occurs. Examples of such dual relationships include, but are not limited to, business or close personal relationships with students, employees, or supervisees. Provision of therapy to students, employees, or supervisees is prohibited. Sexual intimacy with students or supervisees is prohibited.

4.2   Marriage and family therapists do not permit students, employees, or supervisees to perform or to hold themselves out as competent to perform professional services beyond their training, level of experience, and competence.

4.3   Marriage and family therapists do not disclose supervisee confidences except: (a) as mandated by law; (b) to prevent a clear and immediate danger to a person or persons; (c) where the therapist is a defendant in a civil, criminal, or disciplinary action arising from the supervision (in which case supervisee confidences may be disclosed only in the course of that action); (d) in educational or training settings where there are multiple supervisors, and then only to other professional colleagues who share responsibility for the training of the supervisee; or (e) if there is a waiver previously obtained in writing, and then such information may be revealed only in accordance with the terms of the waiver.

5.   RESPONSIBILITY TO RESEARCH PARTICIPANTS

Investigators respect the dignity and protect the welfare of participants in research and are aware of federal and state laws and regulations and professional standards governing the conduct of research.

5.1   Investigators are responsible for making careful examinations of ethical acceptability in planning studies. To the extent that services to research participants may be compromised by participation in research, investigators seek the ethical advice of qualified professionals not directly involved in the investigation and observe safeguards to protect the rights of research participants.

5.2   Investigators requesting participants' involvement in research inform them of all aspects of the research that might reasonably be expected to influence willingness to participate. Investigators are especially sensitive to the possibility of diminished consent when participants are also receiving clinical services, have impairments which limit understanding and/or communication, or when participants are children.

5.3   Investigators respect participants' freedom to decline participation in or to withdraw from a research study at any time. This obligation requires special thought and consideration when investigators or other members of the research team are in positions of authority or influence over participants. Marriage and family therapists, therefore, make every effort to avoid dual relationships with research participants that could impair professional judgment or increase the risk of exploitation.

5.4   Information obtained about a research participant during the course of an investigation is confidential unless there is a waiver previously obtained in writing. When the possibility exists that others, including family members, may obtain access to such information, this possibility, together with the plan for protecting confidentiality, is explained as part of the procedure for obtaining informed consent.

6.   RESPONSIBILITY TO THE PROFESSION

Marriage and family therapists respect the rights and responsibilities of professional colleagues and participate in activities which advance the goals of the profession.

6.1   Marriage and family therapists remain accountable to the standards of the profession when acting as members or employees of organizations.

6.2   Marriage and family therapists assign publication credit to those who have contributed to a publication in proportion to their contributions and in accordance with customary professional publication practices.

6.3   Marriage and family therapists who are the authors of books or other materials that are published or distributed cite persons to whom credit for original ideas is due.

6.4   Marriage and family therapists who are the authors of books or other materials published or distributed by an organization take reasonable precautions to ensure that the organization promotes and advertises the materials accurately and factually.

6.5   Marriage and family therapists participate in activities that contribute to a better community and society, including devoting a portion of their professional activity to services for which there is little or no financial return.

6.6   Marriage and family therapists are concerned with developing laws and regulations pertaining to marriage and family therapy that serve the public interest, and with altering such laws and regulations that are not in the public interest.

6.7   Marriage and family therapists encourage public participation in the design and delivery of professional services and in the regulation of practitioners.

7.   FINANCIAL ARRANGEMENTS

Marriage and family therapists make financial arrangements with clients, third party payors, and supervisees that are reasonably understandable and conform to accepted professional practices.

7.1   Marriage and family therapists do not offer or accept payment for referrals.

7.2   Marriage and family therapists do not charge excessive fees for services.

7.3 Marriage and family therapists disclose their fees to clients and supervisees at the beginning of services.

7.4 Marriage and family therapists represent facts truthfully to clients, third party payors, and supervisees regarding services rendered.

8. ADVERTISING

Marriage and family therapists engage in appropriate informational activities, including those that enable laypersons to choose professional services on an informed basis.

General Advertising

8.1 Marriage and family therapists accurately represent their competence, education, training, and experience relevant to their practice of marriage and family therapy.

8.2 Marriage and family therapists assure that advertisements and publications in any media (such as directories, announcements, business cards, newspapers, radio, television, and facsimiles) convey information that is necessary for the public to make an appropriate selection of professional services. Information could include: (a) office information, such as name, address, telephone number, credit card acceptability, fees, languages spoken, and office hours; (b) appropriate degrees, state licensure and/or certification, and AAMFT Clinical Member status; and (c) description of practice. (For requirements for advertising under the AAMFT name, logo, and/or the abbreviated initials AAMFT, see Subprinciple 8.15, below).

8.3 Marriage and family therapists do not use a name which could mislead the public concerning the identity, responsibility, source, and status of those practicing under that name and do not hold themselves out as being partners or associates of a firm if they are not.

8.4 Marriage and family therapists do not use any professional identification (such as a business card, office sign, letterhead, or telephone or association directory listing) if it includes a statement or claim that is false, fraudulent, misleading, or deceptive. A statement is false, fraudulent, misleading, or deceptive if it (a) contains a material misrepresentation of fact; (b) fails to state any material fact necessary to make the statement, in light of all circumstances, not misleading; or (c) is intended to or is likely to create an unjustified expectation.

8.5   Marriage and family therapists correct, wherever possible, false, misleading, or inaccurate information and representations made by others concerning the therapist's qualifications, services, or products.

8.6   Marriage and family therapists make certain that the qualifications of persons in their employ are represented in a manner that is not false, misleading, or deceptive.

8.7   Marriage and family therapists may represent themselves as specializing within a limited area of marriage and family therapy, but only if they have the education and supervised experience in settings which meet recognized professional standards to practice in that specialty area.

Advertising Using AAMFT Designations

8.8   The AAMFT designations of Clinical Member, Approved Supervisor, and Fellow may be used in public information or advertising materials only by persons holding such designations. Persons holding such designations may, for example, advertise in the following manner:

   - *Jane Doe, Ph.D., a Clinical Member of the American Association for Marriage and Family Therapy.*
   Alternately, the advertisement could read:
   Jane Doe, Ph.D., AAMFT Clinical Member.

   - *John Doe, Ph.D., an Approved Supervisor of the American Association for Marriage and Family Therapy.*

Alternately, the advertisement could read:
John Doe, Ph.D., AAMFT Approved Supervisor.

- *Jane Doe, Ph.D., a Fellow of the American Association for Marriage and Family Therapy.*
Alternately, the advertisement could read:
Jane Doe, Ph.D., AAMFT Fellow.

More than one designation may be used if held by the AAMFT Member.

8.9   Marriage and family therapists who hold the AAMFT Approved Supervisor or the Fellow designation may not represent the designation as an advanced clinical status.

8.10   Student, Associate, and Affiliate Members may not use their AAMFT membership status in public information or advertising materials. Such listings on professional résumés are not considered advertisements.

8.11   Persons applying for AAMFT membership may not list their application status on any résumé or advertisement.

8.12   In conjunction with their AAMFT membership, marriage and family therapists claim as evidence of educational qualifications only those degrees (a) from regionally accredited institutions or (b) from institutions recognized by states which license or certify marriage and family therapists, but only if such state regulation is recognized by AAMFT.

8.13   Marriage and family therapists may not use the initials AAMFT following their name in the manner of an academic degree.

8.14   Marriage and family therapists may not use the AAMFT name, logo, and/or the abbreviated initials AAMFT or make any other such representation which would imply that they speak for or represent the Association. The Association is the sole owner of its name, logo, and the abbreviated initials

AAMFT. Its committees and divisions, operating as such, may use the name, logo, and/or the abbreviated initials, AAMFT, in accordance with AAMFT policies.

8.15   Authorized advertisements of Clinical Members under the AAMFT name, logo, and/or the abbreviated initials AAMFT may include the following: the Clinical Member's name, degree, license or certificate held when required by state law, name of business, address, and telephone number. If a business is listed, it must follow, not precede the Clinical Member's name. Such listings may not include AAMFT offices held by the Clinical Member, nor any specializations, since such a listing under the AAMFT name, logo, and/or the abbreviated initials, AAMFT, would imply that this specialization has been credentialed by AAMFT.

8.16   Marriage and family therapists use their membership in AAMFT only in connection with their clinical and professional activities.

8.17   Only AAMFT divisions and programs accredited by the AAMFT Commission on Accreditation for Marriage and Family Therapy Education, not businesses nor organizations, may use any AAMFT-related designation or affiliation in public information or advertising materials, and then only in accordance with AAMFT policies.

8.18   Programs accredited by the AAMFT Commission on Accreditation for Marriage and Family Therapy Education may not use the AAMFT name, logo, and/or the abbreviated initials, AAMFT. Instead, they may have printed on their stationery and other appropriate materials a statement such as:

The (name of program) *of the* (name of institution) *is accredited by the AAMFT Commission on Accreditation for Marriage and Family Therapy Education.*

8.19   Programs not accredited by the AAMFT Commission on Accreditation for Marriage and Family Therapy Education may not use the AAMFT name, logo, and/or the abbreviated initials, AAMFT. They may not state in printed program materials, program advertisements, and student advisement that their courses and training opportunities are accepted by AAMFT to meet AAMFT membership requirements.

Appendix B

The Principles of Medical Ethics
With Annotations Especially
Applicable to Psychiatry
American Psychiatric Association*

In 1973, the American Psychiatric Association published the first edition of THE PRINCIPLES OF MEDICAL ETHICS WITH ANNOTATIONS ESPECIALLY APPLICABLE TO PSYCHIATRY. Subsequently, revisions were published as the Board of Trustees and the Assembly approved additional annotations. In July of 1980, the American Medical Association approved a new version of the Principles of Medical Ethics (the first revision since 1957) and the APA Ethics Committee[1] incorporated many of its annotations into the new Principles, which resulted in the 1981 edition and subsequent revisions.

FOREWORD

All physicians should practice in accordance with the medical code of ethics set forth in the Principles of Medical Ethics of the American Medical Association. An up-to-date expression and elaboration of these statements is found in the Opinions and Reports of the Council on

---

*Note: From *The Principles of Medical Ethics With Annotations Especially Applicable to Psychiatry.* Copyright © 1993 by the American Psychiatric Association. Reprinted by permission of the American Psychiatric Association.

[1]The committee included Herbert Klemmer, M.D., Chairperson, Miltiades Zaphiropoulos, M.D., Ewald Busse, M.D., John R. Saunders, M.D., and Robert McDevitt, M.D. J. Brand Brickman, M.D., William P. Camp, M.D., and Robert A. Moore, M.D. served as consultants to the APA Ethics Committee.

Ethical and Judicial Affairs of the American Medical Association.[2] Psychiatrists are strongly advised to be familiar with these documents.[3]

However, these general guidelines have sometimes been difficult to interpret for psychiatry, so further annotations to the basic principles are offered in this document. While psychiatrists have the same goals as all physicians, there are special ethical problems in psychiatric practice that differ in coloring and degree from ethical problems in other branches of medical practice, even though the basic principles are the same. The annotations are not designed as absolutes and will be revised from time to time so as to be applicable to current practices and problems.

Following are the AMA Principles of Medical Ethics, printed in their entirety, and then each principle printed separately along with an annotation especially applicable to psychiatry.

PRINCIPLES WITH ANNOTATIONS

Following are each of the AMA Principles of Medical Ethics printed separately along with annotations especially applicable to psychiatry.

PREAMBLE

The medical profession has long subscribed to a body of ethical statements developed primarily for the benefit of the patient. As a member of this profession, a physician must recognize responsibility not only to patients but also to society, to other health professionals, and to self. The following Principles, adopted by the American Medical Association, are not laws but standards of conduct, which define the essentials of honorable behavior for the physician.[4]

---

[2]Current Opinions of the Council on Ethical and Judicial Affairs, Chicago, American Medical Association, 1992.

[3]Chapter 8, Section 1 of the Bylaws of the American Psychiatric Association states, "All members of the American Psychiatric Association shall be bound by the ethical code of the medical profession, specifically defined in The Principles of Medical Ethics of the American Medical Association." In interpreting the APA Constitution and Bylaws, it is the opinion of the Board of Trustees that inactive status in no way removes a physician member from responsibility to abide by the Principles of Medical Ethics.

[4]Statements in italics are taken directly from the American Medical Association's Principles of Medical Ethics.

SECTION 1

A physician shall be dedicated to providing competent medical service with compassion and respect for human dignity.

1.   The patient may place his/her trust in his/her psychiatrist knowing that the psychiatrist's ethics and professional responsibilities preclude him/her gratifying his/her own needs by exploiting the patient.   The psychiatrist shall be ever vigilant about the impact that his/her conduct has upon the boundaries of the doctor/patient relationship, and thus upon the well being of the patient.   These requirements become particularly important because of the essentially private, highly personal, and sometimes intensely emotional nature of the relationship established with the psychiatrist.

2.   A psychiatrist should not be a party to any type of policy that excludes, segregates, or demeans the dignity of any patient because of ethnic origin, race, sex, creed, age, socioeconomic status, or sexual orientation.

3.   In accord with the requirements of law and accepted medical practice, it is ethical for a physician to submit his/her work to peer review and to the ultimate authority of the medical staff executive body and the hospital administration and its governing body.   In case of dispute, the ethical psychiatrist has the following steps available:

    a.   Seek appeal from the medical staff decision to a joint conference committee, including members of the medical staff executive committee and the executive committee of the governing board.   At this appeal, the ethical psychiatrist could request that outside opinions be considered.

    b.   Appeal to the governing body itself.

    c.   Appeal to state agencies regulating licensure of hospitals if, in the particular state, they concern themselves with matters of professional competency and quality of care.

    d.   Attempt to educate colleagues through development of research projects and data and presentations at professional meetings and in professional journals.

    e.   Seek redress in local courts, perhaps through an enjoining injunction against the governing body.

    f.   Public education as carried out by an ethical psychiatrist would not utilize appeals based solely upon emotion, but would be presented in a professional way and without any potential exploitation of patients through testimonials.

4.   A psychiatrist should not be a participant in a legally authorized execution.

SECTION 2

A physician shall deal honestly with patients and colleagues, and strive to expose those physicians deficient in character or competence, or who engage in fraud or deception.

1.   The requirement that the physician conduct himself/herself with propriety in his/her profession and in all the actions of his/her life is especially important in the case of the psychiatrist because the patient tends to model his/her behavior after that of his/her psychiatrist by iden-tification. Further, the necessary intensity of the treatment relationship may tend to activate sexual and other needs and fantasies on the part of both patient and psychiatrist, while weakening the objectivity necessary for control. Additionally, the inherent inequality in the doctor-patient relationship may lead to exploitation of the patient. Sexual activity with a current or former patient is unethical.

2.   The psychiatrist should diligently guard against exploiting infor-mation furnished by the patient and should not use the unique position of power afforded him/her by the psychotherapeutic situation to influ-ence the patient in any way not directly relevant to the treatment goals.

3.   A psychiatrist who regularly practices outside his/her area of professional competence should be considered unethical. Determination of professional competence should be made by peer review boards or other appropriate bodies.

4.   Special consideration should be given to those psychiatrists who, because of mental illness, jeopardize the welfare of their patients and their own reputations and practices. It is ethical, even encouraged, for another psychiatrist to intercede in such situations.

5.   Psychiatric services, like all medical services, are dispensed in the context of a contractual arrangement between the patient and the treating physician. The provisions of the contractual arrangement, which are binding on the physician as well as on the patient, should be explic-itly established.

6.   It is ethical for the psychiatrist to make a charge for a missed appointment when this falls within the terms of the specific contractual agreement with the patient. Charging for a missed appointment or for

one not cancelled 24 hours in advance need not, in itself, be considered unethical if a patient is fully advised that the physician will make such a charge. The practice, however, should be resorted to infrequently and always with the utmost consideration for the patient and his/her circumstances.

7. An arrangement in which a psychiatrist provides supervision or administration to other physicians or nonmedical persons for a percentage of their fees or gross income is not acceptable; this would constitute fee-splitting. In a team of practitioners, or a multidisciplinary team, it is ethical for the psychiatrist to receive income for administration, research, education, or consultation. This should be based upon a mutually agreed upon and set fee or salary, open to renegotiation when a change in the time demand occurs. (See also Section 5, Annotations 2, 3, and 4.)

SECTION 3

A physician shall respect the law and also recognize a responsibility to seek changes in those requirements which are contrary to the best interests of the patient.

1. It would seem self-evident that a psychiatrist who is a law-breaker might be ethically unsuited to practice his/her profession. When such illegal activities bear directly upon his/her practice, this would obviously be the case. However, in other instances, illegal activities such as those concerning the right to protest social injustices might not bear on either the image of the psychiatrist or the ability of the specific psychiatrist to treat his/her patient ethically and well. While no committee or board could offer prior assurance that any illegal activity would not be considered unethical, it is conceivable that an individual could violate a law without being guilty of professionally unethical behavior. Physicians lose no right of citizenship on entry into the profession of medicine.

2. Where not specifically prohibited by local laws governing medical practice, the practice of acupuncture by a psychiatrist is not unethical per se. The psychiatrist should have professional competence in the use of acupuncture. Or, if he/she is supervising the use of acupuncture by non-medical individuals, he/she should provide proper medical supervision. (See also Section 5, Annotations 3 and 4.)

SECTION 4

A physician shall respect the rights of patients, of colleagues, and of other health professionals, and shall safeguard patient confidences within the constraints of the law.

1.   Psychiatric records, including even the identification of a person as a patient, must be protected with extreme care.   Confidentiality is essential to psychiatric treatment.   This is based in part on the special nature of psychiatric therapy as well as on the traditional ethical relationship between physician and patient.   Growing concern regarding the civil rights of patients and the possible adverse effects of computerization, duplication equipment, and data banks makes the dissemination of confidential information an increasing hazard.   Because of the sensitive and private nature of the information with which the psychiatrist deals, he/she must be circumspect in the information that he/she chooses to disclose to others about a patient.   The welfare of the patient must be a continuing consideration.

2.   A psychiatrist may release confidential information only with the authorization of the patient or under proper legal compulsion.   The continuing duty of the psychiatrist to protect the patient includes fully apprising him/her of the connotations of waiving the privilege of privacy.   This may become an issue when the patient is being investigated by a government agency, is applying for a position, or is involved in legal action.   The same principles apply to the release of information concerning treatment to medical departments of government agencies, business organizations, labor unions, and insurance companies.   Information gained in confidence about patients seen in student health services should not be released without the students' explicit permission.

3.   Clinical and other materials used in teaching and writing must be adequately disguised in order to preserve the anonymity of the individuals involved.

4.   The ethical responsibility of maintaining confidentiality holds equally for the consultations in which the patient may not have been present and in which the consultee was not a physician.   In such instances, the physician consultant should alert the consultee to his/her duty of confidentiality.

5.   Ethically the psychiatrist may disclose only that information which is relevant to a given situation.   He/she should avoid offering

speculation as fact. Sensitive information such as an individual's sexual orientation or fantasy material is usually unnecessary.

6.   Psychiatrists are often asked to examine individuals for security purposes, to determine suitability for various jobs, and to determine legal competence. The psychiatrist must fully describe the nature and purpose and lack of confidentiality of the examination to the examinee at the beginning of the examination.

7.   Careful judgment must be exercised by the psychiatrist in order to include, when appropriate, the parents or guardian in the treatment of a minor. At the same time, the psychiatrist must assure the minor proper confidentiality.

8.   Psychiatrists at times may find it necessary, in order to protect the patient or the community from imminent danger, to reveal confidential information disclosed by the patient.

9.   When the psychiatrist is ordered by the court to reveal the confidences entrusted to him/her by patients, he/she may comply or he/she may ethically hold the right to dissent within the framework of the law. When the psychiatrist is in doubt, the right of the patient to confidentiality and, by extension, to unimpaired treatment, should be given priority. The psychiatrist should reserve the right to raise the question of adequate need for disclosure. In the event that the necessity for legal disclosure is demonstrated by the court, the psychiatrist may request the right to disclosure of only that information which is relevant to the legal question at hand.

10. With regard for the person's dignity and privacy and with truly informed consent, it is ethical to present a patient to a scientific gathering, if the confidentiality of the presentation is understood and accepted by the audience.

11. It is ethical to present a patient or former patient to a public gathering or to the news media only if the patient is fully informed of enduring loss of confidentiality, is competent, and consents in writing without coercion.

12. When involved in funded research, the ethical psychiatrist will advise human subjects of the funding source, retain his/her freedom to reveal data and results, and follow all appropriate and current guidelines relative to human subject protection.

13. Ethical considerations in medical practice preclude the psychiatric evaluation of any person charged with criminal acts prior to access to, or availability of, legal counsel. The only exception is the rendering of care to the person for the sole purpose of medical treatment.

14. Sexual involvement between a faculty member or supervisor and a trainee or student, in those situations in which an abuse of power can occur, often takes advantage of inequalities in the working relationship and may be unethical because: (a) any treatment of a patient being supervised may be deleteriously affected; (b) it may damage the trust relationship between teacher and student; and (c) teachers are important professional role models for their trainees and affect their trainees' future professional behavior.

SECTION 5

A physician shall continue to study, apply, and advance scientific knowledge, make relevant information available to patients, colleagues, and the public, obtain consultation, and use the talents of other health professionals when indicated.

1.   Psychiatrists are responsible for their own continuing education and should be mindful of the fact that theirs must be a lifetime of learning.

2.   In the practice of his/her specialty, the psychiatrist consults, associates, collaborates, or integrates his/her work with that of many professionals, including psychologists, psychometricians, social workers, alcoholism counselors, marriage counselors, public health nurses, etc. Furthermore, the nature of modern psychiatric practice extends his/her contacts to such people as teachers, juvenile and adult probation officers, attorneys, welfare workers, agency volunteers, and neighborhood aides. In referring patients for treatment, counseling, or rehabilitation to any of these practitioners, the psychiatrist should ensure that the allied professional or paraprofessional with whom he/she is dealing is a recognized member of his/her own discipline and is competent to carry out the therapeutic task required. The psychiatrist should have the same attitude toward members of the medical profession to whom he/she refers patients. Whenever he/she has reason to doubt the training, skill, or ethical qualifications of the allied professional, the psychiatrist should not refer cases to him/her.

3.   When the psychiatrist assumes a collaborative or supervisory role with another mental health worker, he/she must expend sufficient time to assure that proper care is given. It is contrary to the interests of the patient and to patient care if he/she allows himself/herself to be used as a figurehead.

4.   In relationships between psychiatrists and practicing licensed psychologists, the physician should not delegate to the psychologist or, in fact, to any nonmedical person any matter requiring the exercise of professional medical judgment.

5.   The psychiatrist should agree to the request of a patient for consultation or to such a request from the family of an incompetent or minor patient. The psychiatrist may suggest possible consultants, but the patient or family should be given free choice of the consultant. If the psychiatrist disapproves of the professional qualifications of the consultant or if there is a difference of opinion that the primary therapist cannot resolve, he/she may, after suitable notice, withdraw from the case. If this disagreement occurs within an institution or agency framework, the differences should be resolved by the mediation or arbitration of higher professional authority within the institution or agency.

SECTION 6

A physician shall, in the provision of appropriate patient care, except in emergencies, be free to choose whom to serve, with whom to associate, and the environment in which to provide medical services.

1.   Physicians generally agree that the doctor-patient relationship is such a vital factor in effective treatment of the patient that preservation of optimal conditions for development of a sound working relationship between a doctor and his/her patient should take precedence over all other considerations. Professional courtesy may lead to poor psychiatric care for physicians and their families because of embarrassment over the lack of a complete give-and-take contract.

2.   An ethical psychiatrist may refuse to provide psychiatric treatment to a person who, in the psychiatrist's opinion, cannot be diagnosed as having a mental illness amenable to psychiatric treatment.

SECTION 7

A physician shall recognize a responsibility to participate in activities contributing to an improved community.

1.   Psychiatrists should foster the cooperation of those legitimately concerned with the medical, psychological, social, and legal aspects of mental health and illness. Psychiatrists are encouraged to serve society by advising and consulting with the executive, legislative, and judiciary

branches of the government. A psychiatrist should clarify whether he/she speaks as an individual or as a representative of an organization. Furthermore, psychiatrists should avoid cloaking their public statements with the authority of the profession (e.g., "Psychiatrists know that . . .").

2. Psychiatrists may interpret and share with the public their expertise in the various psychosocial issues that may affect mental health and illness. Psychiatrists should always be mindful of their separate roles as dedicated citizens and as experts in psychological medicine.

3. On occasion psychiatrists are asked for an opinion about an individual who is in the light of public attention, or who has disclosed information about himself/herself through public media. It is unethical for a psychiatrist to offer a professional opinion unless he/she has conducted an examination and has been granted proper authorization for such a statement.

4. The psychiatrist may permit his/her certification to be used for the involuntary treatment of any person only following his/her personal examination of that person. To do so, he/she must find that the person, because of mental illness, cannot form a judgment as to what is in his/her own best interests and that, without such treatment, substantial impairment is likely to occur to the person or others.

Appendix C

Ethical Principles of Psychologists and Code of Conduct
American Psychological Association*

PREAMBLE

Psychologists work to develop a valid and reliable body of scientific knowledge based on research. They may apply that knowledge to human behavior in a variety of contexts. In doing so, they perform many roles, such as researcher, educator, diagnostician, therapist, supervisor, consultant, administrator, social interventionist, and expert witness. Their goal is to broaden knowledge of behavior and, where appropriate, to apply it pragmatically to improve the condition of both the individual and society. Psychologists respect the central importance of freedom of inquiry and expression in research, teaching, and publication. They also

---

*Note: From "Ethical Principles of Psychologists and Code of Conduct" by American Psychological Association, 1992, *American Psychologist, 47*(12), pp. 1597-1611. Copyright © 1992 by American Psychological Association. Reprinted by permission of the American Psychological Association.

This version of the APA Ethics Code was adopted by the American Psychological Association's Council of Representatives during its meeting, August 13 and 16, 1992, and is effective beginning December 1, 1992. Inquiries concerning the substance or interpretation of the American Psychological Association Ethics Code should be addressed to the Director, Office of Ethics, American Psychological Association, 750 First Street, NE, Washington, DC 20002-4242.

This Code will be used to adjudicate complaints brought concerning alleged conduct occurring on or after the effective date. Complaints regarding conduct occurring prior to the effective date will be adjudicated on the basis of the version of the Code that was in effect at the time the conduct occurred, except that no provisions repealed in June 1989, will be enforced even if an earlier version contains the provision. The Ethics Code will undergo continuing review and study for future revisions; comments on the Code may be sent to the above address.

strive to help the public in developing informed judgments and choices concerning human behavior. This Ethics Code provides a common set of values upon which psychologists build their professional and scientific work.

This Code is intended to provide both the general principles and the decision rules to cover most situations encountered by psychologists. It has as its primary goal the welfare and protection of the individuals and groups with whom psychologists work. It is the individual responsibility of each psychologist to aspire to the highest possible standards of conduct. Psychologists respect and protect human and civil rights, and do not knowingly participate in or condone unfair discriminatory practices.

The development of a dynamic set of ethical standards for a psychologist's work-related conduct requires a personal commitment to a lifelong effort to act ethically; to encourage ethical behavior by students, supervisees, employees, and colleagues, as appropriate; and to consult with others, as needed, concerning ethical problems. Each psychologist supplements, but does not violate, the Ethics Code's values and rules on the basis of guidance drawn from personal values, culture, and experience.

GENERAL PRINCIPLES

Principle A: Competence

Psychologists strive to maintain high standards of competence in their work. They recognize the boundaries of their particular competencies and the limitations of their expertise. They provide only those services and use only those techniques for which they are qualified by education, training, or experience. Psychologists are cognizant of the fact that the competencies required in serving, teaching, and/or studying groups of people vary with the distinctive characteristics of those groups. In those areas in which recognized professional standards do not yet exist, psychologists exercise careful judgment and take appropriate precautions to protect the welfare of those with whom they work. They maintain knowledge of relevant scientific and professional information related to the services they render, and they recognize the need for ongoing education. Psychologists make appropriate use of scientific, professional, technical, and administrative resources.

Principle B: Integrity

Psychologists seek to promote integrity in the science, teaching, and practice of psychology. In these activities psychologists are honest, fair, and respectful of others. In describing or reporting their qualifications, services, products, fees, research, or teaching, they do not make statements that are false, misleading, or deceptive. Psychologists strive to be aware of their own belief systems, values, needs, and limitations and the effect of these on their work. To the extent feasible, they attempt to clarify for relevant parties the roles they are performing and to function appropriately in accordance with those roles. Psychologists avoid improper and potentially harmful dual relationships.

Principle C: Professional and Scientific Responsibility

Psychologists uphold professional standards of conduct, clarify their professional roles and obligations, accept appropriate responsibility for their behavior, and adapt their methods to the needs of different populations. Psychologists consult with, refer to, or cooperate with other professionals and institutions to the extent needed to serve the best interests of their patients, clients, or other recipients of their services. Psychologists' moral standards and conduct are personal matters to the same degree as is true for any other person, except as psychologists' conduct may compromise their professional responsibilities or reduce the public's trust in psychology and psychologists. Psychologists are concerned about the ethical compliance of their colleagues' scientific and professional conduct. When appropriate, they consult with colleagues in order to prevent or avoid unethical conduct.

Principle D: Respect for People's Rights and Dignity

Psychologists accord appropriate respect to the fundamental rights, dignity, and worth of all people. They respect the rights of individuals to privacy, confidentiality, self-determination, and autonomy, mindful that legal and other obligations may lead to inconsistency and conflict with the exercise of these rights. Psychologists are aware of cultural, individual, and role differences, including those due to age, gender, race, ethnicity, national origin, religion, sexual orientation, disability, language, and socioeconomic status. Psychologists try to eliminate the effect on their work of biases based on those factors, and they do not knowingly participate in or condone unfair discriminatory practices.

Principle E: Concern for Others' Welfare

Psychologists seek to contribute to the welfare of those with whom they interact professionally. In their professional actions, psychologists weigh the welfare and rights of their patients or clients, students, supervisees, human research participants, and other affected persons, and the welfare of animal subjects of research. When conflicts occur among psychologists' obligations or concerns, they attempt to resolve these conflicts and to perform their roles in a responsible fashion that avoids or minimizes harm. Psychologists are sensitive to real and ascribed differences in power between themselves and others, and they do not exploit or mislead other people during or after professional relationships.

Principle F: Social Responsibility

Psychologists are aware of their professional and scientific responsibilities to the community and the society in which they work and live. They apply and make public their knowledge of psychology in order to contribute to human welfare. Psychologists are concerned about and work to mitigate the causes of human suffering. When undertaking research, they strive to advance human welfare and the science of psychology. Psychologists try to avoid misuse of their work. Psychologists comply with the law and encourage the development of law and social policy that serve the interests of their patients and clients and the public. They are encouraged to contribute a portion of their professional time for little or no personal advantage.

ETHICAL STANDARDS

1.   General Standards

These General Standards are potentially applicable to the professional and scientific activities of all psychologists.

1.01 *Applicability of the Ethics Code*

The activity of a psychologist subject to the Ethics Code may be reviewed under these Ethical Standards only if the activity is part of his or her work-related functions or the activity is psychological in nature. Personal activities having no connection to or effect on psychological roles are not subject to the Ethics Code.

1.02 *Relationship of Ethics and Law*

If psychologists' ethical responsibilities conflict with law, psychologists make known their commitment to the Ethics Code and take steps to resolve the conflict in a responsible manner.

1.03 *Professional and Scientific Relationship*

Psychologists provide diagnostic, therapeutic, teaching, research, supervisory, consultative, or other psychological services only in the context of a defined professional or scientific relationship or role. (See also Standards 2.01, Evaluation, Diagnosis, and Interventions in Professional Context, and 7.02, Forensic Assessments.)

1.04 *Boundaries of Competence*

(a) Psychologists provide services, teach, and conduct research only within the boundaries of their competence, based on their education, training, supervised experience, or appropriate professional experience.

(b) Psychologists provide services, teach, or conduct research in new areas or involving new techniques only after first undertaking appropriate study, training, supervision, and/or consultation from persons who are competent in those areas or techniques.

(c) In those emerging areas in which generally recognized standards for preparatory training do not yet exist, psychologists nevertheless take reasonable steps to ensure the competence of their work and to protect patients, clients, students, research participants, and others from harm.

1.05 *Maintaining Expertise*

Psychologists who engage in assessment, therapy, teaching, research, organizational consulting, or other professional activities maintain a reasonable level of awareness of current scientific and professional information in their fields of activity, and undertake ongoing efforts to maintain competence in the skills they use.

1.06   *Basis for Scientific and Professional Judgments*

Psychologists rely on scientifically and professionally derived knowledge when making scientific or professional judgments or when engaging in scholarly or professional endeavors.

1.07   *Describing the Nature and Results of Psychological Services*

(a) When psychologists provide assessment, evaluation, treatment, counseling, supervision, teaching, consultation, research, or other psychological services to an individual, a group, or an organization, they provide, using language that is reasonably understandable to the recipient of those services, appropriate information beforehand about the nature of such services and appropriate information later about results and conclusions. (See also Standard 2.09, Explaining Assessment Results.)

(b) If psychologists will be precluded by law or by organizational roles from providing such information to particular individuals or groups, they so inform those individuals or groups at the outset of the service.

1.08   *Human Differences*

Where differences of age, gender, race, ethnicity, national origin, religion, sexual orientation, disability, language, or socioeconomic status significantly affect psychologists' work concerning particular individuals or groups, psychologists obtain the training, experience, consultation, or supervision necessary to ensure the competence of their services, or they make appropriate referrals.

1.09   *Respecting Others*

In their work-related activities, psychologists respect the rights of others to hold values, attitudes, and opinions that differ from their own,

1.10   *Nondiscrimination*

In their work-related activities, psychologists do not engage in unfair discrimination based on age, gender, race, ethnicity, national origin, religion, sexual orientation, disability, socioeconomic status, or any basis proscribed by law.

1.11   *Sexual Harassment*

(a) Psychologists do not engage in sexual harassment. Sexual harassment is sexual solicitation, physical advances, or verbal or nonverbal conduct that is sexual in nature, that occurs in connection with the psychologist's activities or roles as a psychologist, and that either: (1) is unwelcome, is offensive, or creates a hostile workplace environment, and the psychologist knows or is told this; or (2) is sufficiently severe or intense to be abusive to a reasonable person in the context. Sexual harassment can consist of a single intense or severe act or of multiple persistent or pervasive acts.

(b) Psychologists accord sexual-harassment complainants and respondents dignity and respect. Psychologists do not participate in denying a person academic admittance or advancement, employment, tenure, or promotion, based solely upon their having made, or their being the subject of, sexual-harassment charges. This does not preclude taking action based upon the outcome of such proceedings or consideration of other appropriate information.

1.12   *Other Harassment*

Psychologists do not knowingly engage in behavior that is harassing or demeaning to persons with whom they interact in their work based on factors such as those persons' age, gender, race, ethnicity, national origin, religion, sexual orientation, disability, language, or socioeconomic status.

1.13   *Personal Problems and Conflicts*

(a) Psychologists recognize that their personal problems and conflicts may interfere with their effectiveness. Accordingly, they refrain from undertaking an activity when they know or should know that their personal problems are likely to lead to harm to a patient, client, colleague, student, research participant, or other person to whom they may owe a professional or scientific obligation.

(b) In addition, psychologists have an obligation to be alert to signs of, and to obtain assistance for, their personal problems at an early stage, in order to prevent significantly impaired performance.

(c) When psychologists become aware of personal problems that may interfere with their performing work-related duties adequately, they take appropriate measures, such as obtaining professional consultation or assistance, and determine whether they should limit, suspend, or terminate their work-related duties.

1.14 *Avoiding Harm*

Psychologists take reasonable steps to avoid harming their patients or clients, research participants, students, and others with whom they work, and to minimize harm where it is foreseeable and unavoidable.

1.15 *Misuse of Psychologists' Influence*

Because psychologists' scientific and professional judgments and actions may affect the lives of others, they are alert to and guard against personal, financial, social, organizational, or political factors that might lead to misuse of their influence.

1.16 *Misuse of Psychologists' Work*

(a) Psychologists do not participate in activities in which it appears likely that their skills or data will be misused by others, unless corrective mechanisms are available. (See also Standard 7.04, Truthfulness and Candor.)

(b) If psychologists learn of misuse or misrepresentation of their work, they take reasonable steps to correct or minimize the misuse or misrepresentation.

1.17 *Multiple Relationships*

(a) In many communities and situations, it may not be feasible or reasonable for psychologists to avoid social or other nonprofessional contacts with persons such as patients, clients, students, supervisees, or research participants. Psychologists must always be sensitive to the potential harmful effects of other contacts on their work and on those persons with whom they deal. A psychologist refrains from entering into or promising another personal, scientific, professional, financial, or other relationship with such persons if it appears likely that such a relationship reasonably might impair the psychologist's objectivity or otherwise interfere with the psychologist's effectively performing his or her functions as a psychologist, or might harm or exploit the other party.

(b) Likewise, whenever feasible, a psychologist refrains from taking on professional or scientific obligations when preexisting relationships would create a risk of such harm.

(c) If a psychologist finds that, due to unforeseen factors, a potentially harmful multiple relationship has arisen, the psychologist attempts to resolve it with due regard for the best interests of the affected person and maximal compliance with the Ethics Code.

1.18 *Barter (With Patients or Clients)*

Psychologists ordinarily refrain from accepting goods, services, or other nonmonetary remuneration from patients or clients in return for psychological services because such arrangements create inherent potential for conflicts, exploitation, and distortion of the professional relationship. A psychologist may participate in bartering *only* if (1) it is not clinically contraindicated, *and* (2) the relationship is not exploitative. (See also Standards 1.17, Multiple Relationships, and 1.25, Fees and Financial Arrangements.)

1.19 *Exploitative Relationships*

(a) Psychologists do not exploit persons over whom they have supervisory, evaluative, or other authority such as students, supervisees, employees, research participants, and clients or patients. (See also Standards 4.05-4.07 regarding sexual involvement with clients or patients.)

(b) Psychologists do not engage in sexual relationships with students or supervisees in training over whom the psychologist has evaluative or direct authority, because such relationships are so likely to impair judgment or be exploitative.

1.20 *Consultations and Referrals*

(a) Psychologists arrange for appropriate consultations and referrals based principally on the best interests of their patients or clients, with appropriate consent, and subject to other relevant considerations, including applicable law and contractual obligations. (See also Standards 5.01, Discussing the Limits of Confidentiality, and 5.06, Consultations.)

(b) When indicated and professionally appropriate, psychologists cooperate with other professionals in order to serve their patients or clients effectively and appropriately.

(c) Psychologists' referral practices are consistent with law.

1.21 *Third-Party Requests for Services*

(a) When a psychologist agrees to provide services to a person or entity at the request of a third party, the psychologist clarifies to the extent feasible, at the outset of the service, the nature of the relationship with each party. This clarification includes the role of the psychologist (such as therapist, organizational consultant, diagnostician, or expert witness), the probable uses of the services provided or the information obtained, and the fact that there may be limits to confidentiality.

(b) If there is a foreseeable risk of the psychologist's being called upon to perform conflicting roles because of the involvement of a third party, the psychologist clarifies the nature and direction of his or her responsibilities, keeps all parties appropriately informed as matters develop, and resolves the situation in accordance with this Ethics Code.

1.22 *Delegation to and Supervision of Subordinates*

(a) Psychologists delegate to their employees, supervisees, and research assistants only those responsibilities that such persons can reasonably be expected to perform competently, on the basis of their education, training, or experience, either independently or with the level of supervision being provided.

(b) Psychologists provide proper training and supervision to their employees or supervisees and take reasonable steps to see that such persons perform services responsibly, competently, and ethically.

(c) If institutional policies, procedures, or practices prevent fulfillment of this obligation, psychologists attempt to modify their role or to correct the situation to the extent feasible.

1.23 *Documentation of Professional and Scientific Work*

(a) Psychologists appropriately document their professional and scientific work in order to facilitate provision of services later by them or by other professionals, to ensure accountability, and to meet other requirements of institutions or the law.

(b) When psychologists have reason to believe that records of their professional services will be used in legal proceedings involving recipients of or participants in their work, they have a responsibility to create and maintain documentation in the kind of detail and quality that would be consistent with reasonable scrutiny in an adjudicative forum. (See also Standard 7.01, Professionalism, under Forensic Activities.)

1.24 Records and Data

Psychologists create, maintain, disseminate, store, retain, and dispose of records and data relating to their research, practice, and other work in accordance with law and in a manner that permits compliance with the requirements of this Ethics Code. (See also Standard 5.04, Maintenance of Records.)

1.25 Fees and Financial Arrangements

(a) As early as is feasible in a professional or scientific relationship, the psychologist and the patient, client, or other appropriate recipient of psychological services reach an agreement specifying the compensation and the billing arrangements.

(b) Psychologists do not exploit recipients of services or payors with respect to fees.

(c) Psychologists' fee practices are consistent with law.

(d) Psychologists do not misrepresent their fees.

(e) If limitations to services can be anticipated because of limitations in financing, this is discussed with the patient, client, or other appropriate recipient of services as early as is feasible. (See also Standard 4.08, Interruption of Services.)

(f) If the patient, client, or other recipient of services does not pay for services as agreed, and if the psychologist wishes to use collection agencies or legal measures to collect the fees, the psychologist first informs the person that such measures will be taken and provides that person an opportunity to make prompt payment. (See also Standard 5.11, Withholding Records for Nonpayment.)

1.26 Accuracy in Reports to Payors and Funding Sources

In their reports to payors for services or sources of research funding, psychologists accurately state the nature of the research or service provided, the fees or charges, and where applicable, the identity of the provider, the findings, and the diagnosis. (See also Standard 5.05, Disclosures.)

1.27 *Referrals and Fees*

When a psychologist pays, receives payment from, or divides fees with another professional other than in an employer-employee relationship, the payment to each is based on the services (clinical, consultative, administrative, or other) provided and is not based on the referral itself.

2.   Evaluation, Assessment, or Intervention

2.01 *Evaluation, Diagnosis, and Interventions in Professional Context*

(a) Psychologists perform evaluations, diagnostic services, or interventions only within the context of a defined professional relationship. (See also Standard 1.03, Professional and Scientific Relationship.)

(b) Psychologists' assessments, recommendations, reports, and psychological diagnostic or evaluative statements are based on information and techniques (including personal interviews of the individual when appropriate) sufficient to provide appropriate substantiation for their findings. (See also Standard 7.02, Forensic Assessments.)

2.02 *Competence and Appropriate Use of Assessments and Interventions*

(a) Psychologists who develop, administer, score, interpret, or use psychological assessment techniques, interviews, tests, or instruments do so in a manner and for purposes that are appropriate in light of the research on or evidence of the usefulness and proper application of the techniques.

(b) Psychologists refrain from misuse of assessment techniques, interventions, results, and interpretations and take reasonable steps to prevent others from misusing the information these techniques provide. This includes refraining from releasing raw test results or raw data to persons, other than to patients or clients as appropriate, who are not qualified to use such information. (See also Standards 1.02, Relationship of Ethics and Law, and 1.04, Boundaries of Competence.)

2.03 *Test Construction*

Psychologists who develop and conduct research with tests and other assessment techniques use scientific procedures and current professional knowledge for test design, standardization, validation, reduction or elimination of bias, and recommendations for use.

2.04   *Use of Assessment in General and With Special Populations*

(a) Psychologists who perform interventions or administer, score, interpret, or use assessment techniques are familiar with the reliability, validation, and related standardization or outcome studies of, and proper applications and uses of, the techniques they use.

(b) Psychologists recognize limits to the certainty with which diagnoses, judgments, or predictions can be made about individuals.

(c) Psychologists attempt to identify situations in which particular interventions or assessment techniques or norms may not be applicable or may require adjustment in administration or interpretation because of factors such as individuals' gender, age, race, ethnicity, national origin, religion, sexual orientation, disability, language, or socioeconomic status.

2.05   *Interpreting Assessment Results*

When interpreting assessment results, including automated interpretations, psychologists take into account the various test factors and characteristics of the person being assessed that might affect psychologists' judgments or reduce the accuracy of their interpretations. They indicate any significant reservations they have about the accuracy or limitations of their interpretations.

2.06   *Unqualified Persons*

Psychologists do not promote the use of psychological assessment techniques by unqualified persons. (See also Standard 1.22, Delegation to and Supervision of Subordinates.)

2.07   *Obsolete Tests and Outdated Test Results*

(a) Psychologists do not base their assessment or intervention decisions or recommendations on data or test results that are outdated for the current purpose.

(b) Similarly, psychologists do not base such decisions or recommendations on tests and measures that are obsolete and not useful for the current purpose.

2.08 *Test Scoring and Interpretation Services*

(a) Psychologists who offer assessment or scoring procedures to other professionals accurately describe the purpose, norms, validity, reliability, and applications of the procedures and any special qualifications applicable to their use.

(b) Psychologists select scoring and interpretation services (including automated services) on the basis of evidence of the validity of the program and procedures as well as on other appropriate considerations.

(c) Psychologists retain appropriate responsibility for the appropriate application, interpretation, and use of assessment instruments, whether they score and interpret such tests themselves or use automated or other services.

2.09 *Explaining Assessment Results*

Unless the nature of the relationship is clearly explained to the person being assessed in advance and precludes provision of an explanation of results (such as in some organizational consulting, preemployment or security screenings, and forensic evaluations), psychologists ensure that an explanation of the results is provided using language that is reasonably understandable to the person assessed or to another legally authorized person on behalf of the client. Regardless of whether the scoring and interpretation are done by the psychologist, by assistants, or by automated or other outside services, psychologists take reasonable steps to ensure that appropriate explanations of results are given.

2.10 *Maintaining Test Security*

Psychologists make reasonable efforts to maintain the integrity and security of tests and other assessment techniques consistent with law, contractural obligations, and in a manner that permits compliance with the requirements of this Ethics Code. (See also Standard 1.02, Relationship of Ethics and Law.)

3.   Advertising and Other Public Statements

3.01 *Definition of Public Statements*

Psychologists comply with this Ethics Code in public statements relating to their professional services, products, or publications or to the field of psychology. Public statements include but are not limited to paid or unpaid advertising, brochures, printed matter, directory listings, personal résumés or curricula vitae, interviews or comments for use in media, statements in legal proceedings, lectures and public oral presentations, and published materials.

3.02 *Statements by Others*

(a) Psychologists who engage others to create or place public statements that promote their professional practice, products, or activities retain professional responsibility for such statements.

(b) In addition, psychologists make reasonable efforts to prevent others whom they do not control (such as employers, publishers, sponsors, organizational clients, and representatives of the print or broadcast media) from making deceptive statements concerning psychologists' practice or professional or scientific activities.

(c) If psychologists learn of deceptive statements about their work made by others, psychologists make reasonable efforts to correct such statements.

(d) Psychologists do not compensate employees of press, radio, television, or other communication media in return for publicity in a news item.

(e) A paid advertisement relating to the psychologist's activities must be identified as such, unless it is already apparent from the context.

3.03 *Avoidance of False or Deceptive Statements*

(a) Psychologists do not make public statements that are false, deceptive, misleading, or fraudulent, either because of what they state, convey, or suggest or because of what they omit, concerning their research, practice, or other work activities or those of persons or organizations with which they are affiliated. As examples (and not in limitation) of this standard, psychologists do not make false or deceptive statements concerning (1) their training, experience, or competence; (2) their academic degrees; (3) their credentials; (4) their institutional or association affiliations; (5) their services; (6) the scientific or clinical basis for, or results or degree of success of, their services; (7) their fees; or (8) their publications or research findings. (See also Standards 6.15, Deception in Research, and 6.18, Providing Participants With Information About the Study.)

(b) Psychologists claim as credentials for their psychological work, only degrees that (1) were earned from a regionally accredited educational institution or (2) were the basis for psychology licensure by the state in which they practice.

3.04   *Media Presentations*

When psychologists provide advice or comment by means of public lectures, demonstrations, radio or television programs, prerecorded tapes, printed articles, mailed material, or other media, they take reasonable precautions to ensure that (1) the statements are based on appropriate psychological literature and practice, (2) the statements are otherwise consistent with this Ethics Code, and (3) the recipients of the information are not encouraged to infer that a relationship has been established with them personally.

3.05   *Testimonials*

Psychologists do not solicit testimonials from current psychotherapy clients or patients or other persons who because of their particular circumstances are vulnerable to undue influence.

3.06   *In-Person Solicitation*

Psychologists do not engage, directly or through agents, in uninvited in-person solicitation of business from actual or potential psychotherapy patients or clients or other persons who because of their particular circumstances are vulnerable to undue influence. However, this does not preclude attempting to implement appropriate collateral contacts with significant others for the purpose of benefiting an already engaged therapy patient.

4.   Therapy

4.01   *Structuring the Relationship*

(a) Psychologists discuss with clients or patients as early as is feasible in the therapeutic relationship appropriate issues, such as the nature and anticipated course of therapy, fees, and confidentiality. (See also Standards 1.25, Fees and Financial Arrangements, and 5.01, Discussing the Limits of Confidentiality.)

(b) When the psychologist's work with clients or patients will be supervised, the above discussion includes that fact, and the name of the supervisor, when the supervisor has legal responsibility for the case.

(c) When the therapist is a student intern, the client or patient is informed of that fact.

(d) Psychologists make reasonable efforts to answer patients' questions and to avoid apparent misunderstandings about therapy. Whenever possible, psychologists provide oral and/or written information, using language that is reasonably understandable to the patient or client.

4.02   *Informed Consent to Therapy*

(a) Psychologists obtain appropriate informed consent to therapy or related procedures, using language that is reasonably understandable to participants. The content of informed consent will vary depending on many circumstances; however, informed consent generally implies that the person (1) has the capacity to consent, (2) has been informed of significant information concerning the procedure, (3) has freely and without undue influence expressed consent, and (4) consent has been appropriately documented.

(b) When persons are legally incapable of giving informed consent, psychologists obtain informed permission from a legally authorized person, if such substitute consent is permitted by law.

(c) In addition, psychologists (1) inform those persons who are legally incapable of giving informed consent about the proposed interventions in a manner commensurate with the persons' psychological capacities, (2) seek their assent to those interventions, and (3) consider such persons' preferences and best interests.

4.03   *Couple and Family Relationships*

(a) When a psychologist agrees to provide services to several persons who have a relationship (such as husband and wife or parents and children), the psychologist attempts to clarify at the outset (1) which of the individuals are patients or clients and (2) the relationship the psychologist will have with each person. This clarification includes the role of the psychologist and the probable uses of the services provided or the information obtained. (See also Standard 5.01, Discussing the Limits of Confidentiality.)

(b) As soon as it becomes apparent that the psychologist may be called on to perform potentially conflicting roles (such as marital counselor to husband and wife, and then witness for one party in a divorce proceeding), the psychologist attempts to clarify and adjust, or withdraw from, roles appropriately. (See also Standard 7.03, Clarification of Role, under Forensic Activities.)

4.04   *Providing Mental Health Services to Those Served by Others*

In deciding whether to offer or provide services to those already receiving mental health services elsewhere, psychologists carefully consider the treatment issues and the potential patient's or client's welfare. The psychologist discusses these issues with the patient or client, or another legally authorized person on behalf of the client, in order to minimize the risk of confusion and conflict, consults with the other service providers when appropriate, and proceeds with caution and sensitivity to the therapeutic issues.

4.05   *Sexual Intimacies With Current Patients or Clients*

Psychologists do not engage in sexual intimacies with current patients or clients.

4.06   *Therapy With Former Sexual Partners*

Psychologists do not accept as therapy patients or clients persons with whom they have engaged in sexual intimacies.

4.07   *Sexual Intimacies With Former Therapy Patients*

(a) Psychologists do not engage in sexual intimacies with a former therapy patient or client for at least two years after cessation or termination of professional services.

(b) Because sexual intimacies with a former therapy patient or client are so frequently harmful to the patient or client, and because such intimacies undermine public confidence in the psychology profession and thereby deter the public's use of needed services, psychologists do not engage in sexual intimacies with former therapy patients and clients even after a two-year interval except in the most unusual circumstances. The psychologist who engages in such activity after the two years following cessation or termination of treatment bears the burden of demonstrating that there has been no exploitation, in light of all relevant factors, including (1) the amount of time that has passed since therapy terminated,

(2) the nature and duration of the therapy, (3) the circumstances of termination, (4) the patient's or client's personal history, (5) the patient's or client's current mental status, (6) the likelihood of adverse impact on the patient or client and others, and (7) any statements or actions made by the therapist during the course of therapy suggesting or inviting the possibility of a posttermination sexual or romantic relationship with the patient or client. (See also Standard 1.17, Multiple Relationships.)

4.08 *Interruption of Services*

(a) Psychologists make reasonable efforts to plan for facilitating care in the event that psychological services are interrupted by factors such as the psychologist's illness, death, unavailability, or relocation or by the client's relocation or financial limitations. (See also Standard 5.09, Preserving Records and Data.)

(b) When entering into employment or contractual relationships, psychologists provide for orderly and appropriate resolution of responsibility for patient or client care in the event that the employment or contractual relationship ends, with paramount consideration given to the welfare of the patient or client.

4.09 *Terminating the Professional Relationship*

(a) Psychologists do not abandon patients or clients. (See also Standard 1.25c, under Fees and Financial Arrangements.)

(b) Psychologists terminate a professional relationship when it becomes reasonably clear that the patient or client no longer needs the service, is not benefiting, or is being harmed by continued service.

(c) Prior to termination for whatever reason, except where precluded by the patient's or client's conduct, the psychologist discusses the patient's or client's views and needs, provides appropriate pretermination counseling, suggests alternative service providers as appropriate, and takes other reasonable steps to facilitate transfer of responsibility to another provider if the patient or client needs one immediately.

5. Privacy and Confidentiality

These Standards are potentially applicable to the professional and scientific activities of all psychologists.

5.01   *Discussing the Limits of Confidentiality*

(a) Psychologists discuss with persons and organizations with whom they establish a scientific or professional relationship (including, to the extent feasible, minors and their legal representatives) (1) the relevant limitations on confidentiality, including limitations where applicable in group, marital, and family therapy or in organizational consulting, and (2) the foreseeable uses of the information generated through their services.

(b) Unless it is not feasible or is contraindicated, the discussion of confidentiality occurs at the outset of the relationship and thereafter as new circumstances may warrant.

(c) Permission for electronic recording of interviews is secured from clients and patients.

5.02   *Maintaining Confidentiality*

Psychologists have a primary obligation and take reasonable precautions to respect the confidentiality rights of those with whom they work or consult, recognizing that confidentiality may be established by law, institutional rules, or professional or scientific relationships. (See also Standard 6.26, Professional Reviewers.)

5.03   *Minimizing Intrusions on Privacy*

(a) In order to minimize intrusions on privacy, psychologists include in written and oral reports, consultations, and the like, only information germane to the purpose for which the communication is made.

(b) Psychologists discuss confidential information obtained in clinical or consulting relationships, or evaluative data concerning patients, individual or organizational clients, students, research participants, supervisees, and employees, only for appropriate scientific or professional purposes and only with persons clearly concerned with such matters.

5.04   *Maintenance of Records*

Psychologists maintain appropriate confidentiality in creating, storing, accessing, transferring, and disposing of records under their control, whether these are written, automated, or in any other medium. Psychologists maintain and dispose of records in accordance with law and in a manner that permits compliance with the requirements of this Ethics Code.

5.05 *Disclosures*

(a) Psychologists disclose confidential information without the consent of the individual only as mandated by law, or where permitted by law for a valid purpose, such as (1) to provide needed professional services to the patient or the individual or organizational client, (2) to obtain appropriate professional consultations, (3) to protect the patient or client or others from harm, or (4) to obtain payment for services, in which instance disclosure is limited to the minimum that is necessary to achieve the purpose.

(b) Psychologists also may disclose confidential information with the appropriate consent of the patient or the individual or organizational client (or of another legally authorized person on behalf of the patient or client), unless prohibited by law.

5.06 *Consultations*

When consulting with colleagues, (1) psychologists do not share confidential information that reasonably could lead to the identification of a patient, client, research participant, or other person or organization with whom they have a confidential relationship unless they have obtained the prior consent of the person or organization or the disclosure cannot be avoided, and (2) they share information only to the extent necessary to achieve the purposes of the consultation. (See also Standard 5.02, Maintaining Confidentiality.)

5.07 *Confidential Information in Databases*

(a) If confidential information concerning recipients of psychological services is to be entered into databases or systems of records available to persons whose access has not been consented to by the recipient, then psychologists use coding or other techniques to avoid the inclusion of personal identifiers.

(b) If a research protocol approved by an institutional review board or similar body requires the inclusion of personal identifiers, such identifiers are deleted before the information is made accessible to persons other than those of whom the subject was advised.

(c) If such deletion is not feasible, then before psychologists transfer such data to others or review such data collected by others, they take reasonable steps to determine that appropriate consent of personally identifiable individuals has been obtained.

5.08   *Use of Confidential Information for Didactic or Other Purposes*

(a) Psychologists do not disclose in their writings, lectures, or other public media, confidential, personally identifiable information concerning their patients, individual or organizational clients, students, research participants, or other recipients of their services that they obtained during the course of their work, unless the person or organization has consented in writing or unless there is other ethical or legal authorization for doing so.

(b) Ordinarily, in such scientific and professional presentations, psychologists disguise confidential information concerning such persons or organizations so that they are not individually identifiable to others and so that discussions do not cause harm to subjects who might identify themselves.

5.09   *Preserving Records and Data*

A psychologist makes plans in advance so that confidentiality of records and data is protected in the event of the psychologist's death, incapacity, or withdrawal from the position or practice.

5.10   *Ownership of Records and Data*

Recognizing that ownership of records and data is governed by legal principles, psychologists take reasonable and lawful steps so that records and data remain available to the extent needed to serve the best interests of patients, individual or organizational clients, research participants, or appropriate others.

5.11   *Withholding Records for Nonpayment*

Psychologists may not withhold records under their control that are requested and imminently needed for a patient's or client's treatment solely because payment has not been received, except as otherwise provided by law.

6. Teaching, Training Supervision, Research, and Publishing

6.01 *Design of Education and Training Programs*

Psychologists who are responsible for education and training programs seek to ensure that the programs are competently designed, provide the proper experiences, and meet the requirements for licensure, certification, or other goals for which claims are made by the program.

6.02 *Descriptions of Education and Training Programs*

(a) Psychologists responsible for education and training programs seek to ensure that there is a current and accurate description of the program content, training goals and objectives, and requirements that must be met for satisfactory completion of the program. This information must be made readily available to all interested parties.

(b) Psychologists seek to ensure that statements concerning their course outlines are accurate and not misleading, particularly regarding the subject matter to be covered, bases for evaluating progress, and the nature of course experiences. (See also Standard 3.03, Avoidance of False or Deceptive Statements.)

(c) To the degree to which they exercise control, psychologists responsible for announcements, catalogs, brochures, or advertisements describing workshops, seminars, or other non-degree-granting educational programs ensure that they accurately describe the audience for which the program is intended, the educational objectives, the presenters, and the fees involved.

6.03 *Accuracy and Objectivity in Teaching*

(a) When engaged in teaching or training, psychologists present psychological information accurately and with a reasonable degree of objectivity.

(b) When engaged in teaching or training, psychologists recognize the power they hold over students or supervisees and therefore make reasonable efforts to avoid engaging in conduct that is personally demeaning to students or supervisees. (See also Standards 1.09, Respecting Others, and 1.12, Other Harassment.)

6.04   *Limitation on Teaching*

Psychologists do not teach the use of techniques or procedures that require specialized training, licensure, or expertise, including but not limited to hypnosis, biofeedback, and projective techniques, to individuals who lack the prerequisite training, legal scope of practice, or expertise.

6.05   *Assessing Student and Supervisee Performance*

(a) In academic and supervisory relationships, psychologists establish an appropriate process for providing feedback to students and supervisees.

(b) Psychologists evaluate students and supervisees on the basis of their actual performance on relevant and established program requirements.

6.06   *Planning Research*

(a) Psychologists design, conduct, and report research in accordance with recognized standards of scientific competence and ethical research.

(b) Psychologists plan their research so as to minimize the possibility that results will be misleading.

(c) In planning research, psychologists consider its ethical acceptability under the Ethics Code. If an ethical issue is unclear, psychologists seek to resolve the issue through consultation with institutional review boards, animal care and use committees, peer consultations, or other proper mechanisms.

(d) Psychologists take reasonable steps to implement appropriate protections for the rights and welfare of human participants, other persons affected by the research, and the welfare of animal subjects.

6.07   *Responsibility*

(a) Psychologists conduct research competently and with due concern for the dignity and welfare of the participants.

(b) Psychologists are responsible for the ethical conduct of research conducted by them or by others under their supervision or control.

(c) Researchers and assistants are permitted to perform only those tasks for which they are appropriately trained and prepared.

(d) As part of the process of development and implementation of research projects, psychologists consult those with expertise concerning any special population under investigation or most likely to be affected.

6.08 *Compliance With Law and Standards*

Psychologists plan and conduct research in a manner consistent with federal and state law and regulations, as well as professional standards governing the conduct of research, and particularly those standards governing research with human participants and animal subjects.

6.09 *Institutional Approval*

Psychologists obtain from host institutions or organizations appropriate approval prior to conducting research, and they provide accurate information about their research proposals. They conduct the research in accordance with the approved research protocol.

6.10 *Research Responsibilities*

Prior to conducting research (except research involving only anonymous surveys, naturalistic observations, or similar research), psychologists enter into an agreement with participants that clarifies the nature of the research and the responsibilities of each party.

6.11 *Informed Consent to Research*

(a) Psychologists use language that is reasonably understandable to research participants in obtaining their appropriate informed consent (except as provided in Standard 6.12, Dispensing With Informed Consent). Such informed consent is appropriately documented.

(b) Using language that is reasonably understandable to participants, psychologists inform participants of the nature of the research; they inform participants that they are free to participate or to decline to participate or to withdraw from the research; they explain the foreseeable consequences of declining or withdrawing; they inform participants of significant factors that may be expected to influence their willingness to participate (such as risks, discomfort, adverse effects, or limitations on confidentiality, except as provided in Standard 6.15, Deception in Research); and they explain other aspects about which the prospective participants inquire.

(c) When psychologists conduct research with individuals such as students or subordinates, psychologists take special care to protect the prospective participants from adverse consequences of declining or withdrawing from participation.

(d) When research participation is a course requirement or opportunity for extra credit, the prospective participant is given the choice of equitable alternative activities.

(e) For persons who are legally incapable of giving informed consent, psychologists nevertheless (1) provide an appropriate explanation, (2) obtain the participant's assent, and (3) obtain appropriate permission from a legally authorized person, if such substitute consent is permitted by law.

6.12 *Dispensing With Informed Consent*

Before determining that planned research (such as research involving only anonymous questionnaires, naturalistic observations, or certain kinds of archival research) does not require the informed consent of research participants, psychologists consider applicable regulations and institutional review board requirements, and they consult with colleagues as appropriate.

6.13 *Informed Consent in Research Filming or Recording*

Psychologists obtain informed consent from research participants prior to filming or recording them in any form, unless the research involves simply naturalistic observations in public places and it is not anticipated that the recording will be used in a manner that could cause personal identification or harm.

6.14 *Offering Inducements for Research Participants*

(a) In offering professional services as an inducement to obtain research participants, psychologists make clear the nature of the services, as well as the risks, obligations, and limitations. (See also Standard 1.18, Barter [With Patients or Clients].)

(b) Psychologists do not offer excessive or inappropriate financial or other inducements to obtain research participants, particularly when it might tend to coerce participation.

6.15   *Deception in Research*

(a) Psychologists do not conduct a study involving deception unless they have determined that the use of deceptive techniques is justified by the study's prospective scientific, educational, or applied value and that equally effective alternative procedures that do not use deception are not feasible.

(b) Psychologists never deceive research participants about significant aspects that would affect their willingness to participate, such as physical risks, discomfort, or unpleasant emotional experiences.

(c) Any other deception that is an integral feature of the design and conduct of an experiment must be explained to participants as early as is feasible, preferably at the conclusion of their participation, but no later than at the conclusion of the research. (See also Standard 6.18, Providing Participants With Information About the Study.)

6.16   *Sharing and Utilizing Data*

Psychologists inform research participants of their anticipated sharing or further use of personally identifiable research data and of the possibility of unanticipated future uses.

6.17   *Minimizing Invasiveness*

In conducting research, psychologists interfere with the participants or milieu from which data are collected only in a manner that is warranted by an appropriate research design and that is consistent with psychologists' roles as scientific investigators.

6.18   *Providing Participants With Information About the Study*

(a) Psychologists provide a prompt opportunity for participants to obtain appropriate information about the nature, results, and conclusions of the research, and psychologists attempt to correct any misconceptions that participants may have.

(b) If scientific or humane values justify delaying or withholding this information, psychologists take reasonable measures to reduce the risk of harm.

6.19 *Honoring Commitments*

Psychologists take reasonable measures to honor all commitments they have made to research participants.

6.20 *Care and Use of Animals in Research*

(a) Psychologists who conduct research involving animals treat them humanely.

(b) Psychologists acquire, care for, use, and dispose of animals in compliance with current federal, state, and local laws and regulations, and with professional standards.

(c) Psychologists trained in research methods and experienced in the care of laboratory animals supervise all procedures involving animals and are responsible for ensuring appropriate consideration of their comfort, health, and humane treatment.

(d) Psychologists ensure that all individuals using animals under their supervision have received instruction in research methods and in the care, maintenance, and handling of the species being used, to the extent appropriate to their role.

(e) Responsibilities and activities of individuals assisting in a research project are consistent with their respective competencies.

(f) Psychologists make reasonable efforts to minimize the discomfort, infection, illness, and pain of animal subjects.

(g) A procedure subjecting animals to pain, stress, or privation is used only when an alternative procedure is unavailable and the goal is justified by its prospective scientific, educational, or applied value.

(h) Surgical procedures are performed under appropriate anesthesia; techniques to avoid infection and minimize pain are followed during and after surgery.

(i) When it is appropriate that the animals's life be terminated, it is done rapidly, with an effort to minimize pain, and in accordance with accepted procedures.

6.21 *Reporting of Results*

(a) Psychologists do not fabricate data or falsify results in their publications.

(b) If psychologists discover significant errors in their published data, they take reasonable steps to correct such errors in a correction, retraction, erratum, or other appropriate publication means.

6.22 *Plagiarism*

Psychologists do not present substantial portions or elements of another's work or data as their own, even if the other work or data source is cited occasionally.

6.23 *Publication Credit*

(a) Psychologists take responsibility and credit, including authorship credit, only for work they have actually performed or to which they have contributed.

(b) Principal authorship and other publication credits accurately reflect the relative scientific or professional contributions of the individuals involved, regardless of their relative status. Mere possession of an institutional position, such as Department Chair, does not justify authorship credit. Minor contributions to the research or to the writing for publications are appropriately acknowledged, such as in footnotes or in an introductory statement.

(c) A student is usually listed as principal author on any multiple-authored article that is substantially based on the student's dissertation or thesis.

6.24 *Duplicate Publication of Data*

Psychologists do not publish, as original data, data that have been previously published. This does not preclude republishing data when they are accompanied by proper acknowledgement.

6.25 *Sharing Data*

After research results are published, psychologists do not withhold the data on which their conclusions are based from other competent professionals who seek to verify the substantive claims through reanalysis and who intend to use such data only for that purpose, provided that the confidentiality of the participants can be protected and unless legal rights concerning proprietary data preclude their release.

6.26 *Professional Reviewers*

Psychologists who review material submitted for publication, grant, or other research proposal review respect the confidentiality of and the proprietary rights in such information of those who submitted it.

7.   Forensic Activities

7.01   *Professionalism*

Psychologists who perform forensic functions, such as assessments, interviews, consultations, reports, or expert testimony, must comply with all other provisions of this Ethics Code to the extent that they apply to such activities. In addition, psychologists base their forensic work on appropriate knowledge of and competence in the areas underlying such work, including specialized knowledge concerning special populations. (See also Standards 1.06, Basis for Scientific and Professional Judgments; 1.08, Human Differences; 1.15, Misuse of Psychologists' Influence; and 1.23, Documentation of Professional and Scientific Work.)

7.02   *Forensic Assessments*

(a) Psychologists' forensic assessments, recommendations, and reports are based on information and techniques (including personal interviews of the individual, when appropriate) sufficient to provide appropriate substantiation for their findings. (See also Standards 1.03, Professional and Scientific Relationship; 1.23, Documentation of Professional and Scientific Work; 2.01, Evaluation, Diagnosis, and Interventions in Professional Context; and 2.05, Interpreting Assessment Results.)

(b) Except as noted in (c), below, psychologists provide written or oral forensic reports or testimony of the psychological characteristics of an individual only after they have conducted an examination of the individual adequate to support their statements or conclusions.

(c) When, despite reasonable efforts, such an examination is not feasible, psychologists clarify the impact of their limited information on the reliability and validity of their reports and testimony, and they appropriately limit the nature and extent of their conclusions or recommendations.

7.03   *Clarification of Role*

In most circumstances, psychologists avoid performing multiple and potentially conflicting roles in forensic matters. When psychologists may be called on to serve in more than one role in a legal proceeding - for example, as consultant or expert for one party or for the court and as a fact witness - they clarify role expectations and the extent of confidentiality in advance to the extent feasible, and thereafter as changes occur, in order to avoid compromising their professional judgment and objectivity and in order to avoid misleading others regarding their role.

7.04 *Truthfulness and Candor*

(a) In forensic testimony and reports, psychologists testify truthfully, honestly, and candidly and, consistent with applicable legal procedures, describe fairly the bases for their testimony and conclusions.

(b) Whenever necessary to avoid misleading, psychologists acknowledge the limits of their data or conclusions.

7.05 *Prior Relationships*

A prior professional relationship with a party does not preclude psychologists from testifying as fact witnesses or from testifying to their services to the extent permitted by applicable law. Psychologists appropriately take into account ways in which the prior relationship might affect their professional objectivity or opinions and disclose the potential conflict to the relevant parties.

7.06 *Compliance With Law and Rules*

In performing forensic roles, psychologists are reasonably familiar with the rules governing their roles. Psychologists are aware of the occasionally competing demands placed upon them by these principles and the requirements of the court system, and attempt to resolve these conflicts by making known their commitment to this Ethics Code and taking steps to resolve the conflict in a responsible manner. (See also Standard 1.02, Relationship of Ethics and Law.)

8. Resolving Ethical Issues

8.01 *Familiarity With Ethics Code*

Psychologists have an obligation to be familiar with this Ethics Code, other applicable ethics codes, and their application to psychologists' work. Lack of awareness or misunderstanding of an ethical standard is not itself a defense to a charge of unethical conduct.

8.02 *Confronting Ethical Issues*

When a psychologist is uncertain whether a particular situation or course of action would violate this Ethics Code, the psychologist ordinarily consults with other psychologists knowledgeable about ethical issues, with state or national psychology ethics committees, or with other appropriate authorities in order to choose a proper response.

8.03 *Conflicts Between Ethics and Organizational Demands*

If the demands of an organization with which psychologists are affiliated conflict with this Ethics Code, psychologists clarify the nature of the conflict, make known their commitment to the Ethics Code, and to the extent feasible, seek to resolve the conflict in a way that permits the fullest adherence to the Ethics Code.

8.04 *Informal Resolution of Ethical Violations*

When psychologists believe that there may have been an ethical violation by another psychologist, they attempt to resolve the issue by bringing it to the attention of that individual if an informal resolution appears appropriate and the intervention does not violate any confidentiality rights that may be involved.

8.05 *Reporting Ethical Violations*

If an apparent ethical violation is not appropriate for informal resolution under Standard 8.04 or is not resolved properly in that fashion, psychologists take further action appropriate to the situation, unless such action conflicts with confidentiality rights in ways that cannot be resolved. Such action might include referral to state or national committees on professional ethics or to state licensing boards.

8.06 *Cooperating With Ethics Committees*

Psychologists cooperate in ethics investigations, proceedings, and resulting requirements of the APA or any affiliated state psychological association to which they belong. In doing so, they make reasonable efforts to resolve any issues as to confidentiality. Failure to cooperate is itself an ethics violation.

8.07   *Improper Complaints*

Psychologists do not file or encourage the filing of ethics complaints that are frivolous and are intended to harm the respondent rather than to protect the public.

Appendix D

Code of Ethics
National Association of
Social Workers (NASW)*

PREAMBLE

This code is intended to serve as a guide to the everyday conduct of members of the social work profession and as a basis for the adjudication of issues in ethics when the conduct of social workers is alleged to deviate from the standards expressed or implied in this code. It represents standards of ethical behavior for social workers in professional relationships with those served, with colleagues, with employers, with other individuals and professions, and with the community and society as a whole. It also embodies standards of ethical behavior governing individual conduct to the extent that such conduct is associated with an individual's status and identity as a social worker.

This code is based on the fundamental values of the social work profession that include the worth, dignity, and uniqueness of all persons as well as their rights and opportunities. It is also based on the nature of social work, which fosters conditions that promote these values.

In subscribing to and abiding by this code, the social worker is expected to view ethical responsibility in as inclusive a context as each situation demands and within which ethical judgement is required. The social worker is expected to take into consideration all the principles in this code that have a bearing upon any situation in which ethical judgement is to be exercised and professional intervention or conduct is planned. The course of action that the social worker chooses is expected to be consistent with the spirit as well as the letter of this code.

*Note: From *Code of Ethics of the National Association of Social Workers* (NASW), copyright © 1993, as adopted by the 1979 NASW Delegate Assembly and revised by the 1990 and 1993 NASW Delegate Assembly, Washington, DC: NASW. Reprinted by permission of the NASW.

In itself, this code does not represent a set of rules that will prescribe all the behaviors of social workers in all the complexities of professional life. Rather, it offers general principles to guide conduct, and the judicious appraisal of conduct, in situations that have ethical implications. It provides the basis for making judgements about ethical actions before and after they occur. Frequently, the particular situation determines the ethical principles that apply and the manner of their application. In such cases, not only the particular ethical principles are taken into immediate consideration, but also the entire code and its spirit. Specific applications of ethical principles must be judged within the context in which they are being considered. Ethical behavior in a given situation must satisfy not only the judgement of the individual social worker, but also the judgement of an unbiased jury of professional peers.

This code should not be used as an instrument to deprive any social worker of the opportunity or freedom to practice with complete professional integrity; nor should any disciplinary action be taken on the basis of this code without maximum provision for safeguarding the rights of the social worker affected.

The ethical behavior of social workers results not from edict, but from a personal commitment of the individual. This code is offered to affirm the will and zeal of all social workers to be ethical and to act ethically in all that they do as social workers.

The following codified ethical principles should guide social workers in the various roles and relationships and at the various levels of responsibility in which they function professionally. These principles also serve as a basis for the adjudication by the National Association of Social Workers of issues in ethics.

In subscribing to this code, social workers are required to cooperate in its implementation and abide by any disciplinary rulings based on it. They should also take adequate measures to discourage, prevent, expose, and correct the unethical conduct of colleagues. Finally, social workers should be equally ready to defend and assist colleagues unjustly charged with unethical conduct.

THE NASW CODE OF ETHICS

I. The Social Worker's Conduct and Comportment as a Social Worker
   A. Propriety - The social worker should maintain high standards of personal conduct in the capacity or identity as social worker.

1. The private conduct of the social worker is a personal matter to the same degree as is any other person's, except when such conduct compromises the fulfillment of professional responsibilities.
2. The social worker should not participate in, condone, or be associated with dishonesty, fraud, deceit, or misrepresentation.
3. The social worker should distinguish clearly between statements and actions made as a private individual and as a representative of the social work profession or an organization or group.

B.   Competence and Professional Development - The social worker should strive to become and remain proficient in professional practice and the performance of professional functions.

1. The social worker should accept responsibility or employment only on the basis of existing competence or the intention to acquire the necessary competence.
2. The social worker should not misrepresent professional qualifications, education, experience, or affiliations.
3. The social worker should not allow his or her own personal problems, psychosocial distress, substance abuse, or mental health difficulties to interfere with professional judgement and performance or jeopardize the best interests of those for whom the social worker has a professional responsibility.
4. The social worker whose personal problems, psychosocial distress, substance abuse, or mental health difficulties interfere with professional judgement and performance should immediately seek consultation and take appropriate remedial action by seeking professional help, making adjustments in workload, terminating practice, or taking any other steps necessary to protect clients and others.

C.   Service - The social worker should regard as primary the service obligation of the social work profession.

1. The social worker should retain ultimate responsibility for the quality and extent of the service that individual assumes, assigns, or performs.
2. The social worker should act to prevent practices that are inhumane or discriminatory against any person or group of persons.

D. Integrity - The social worker should act in accordance with the highest standards of professional integrity and impartiality.

1. The social worker should be alert to and resist the influences and pressures that interfere with the exercise of professional discretion and impartial judgement required for the performance of professional functions.

2. The social worker should not exploit professional relationships for personal gain.

E. Scholarship and Research - The social worker engaged in study and research should be guided by the conventions of scholarly inquiry.

1. The social worker engaged in research should consider carefully its possible consequences for human beings.

2. The social worker engaged in research should ascertain that the consent of participants in the research is voluntary and informed, without any implied deprivation or penalty for refusal to participate, and with due regard for participants' privacy and dignity.

3. The social worker engaged in research should protect participants from unwarranted physical or mental discomfort, distress, harm, danger, or deprivation.

4. The social worker who engages in the evaluation of services or cases should discuss them only for the professional purposes and only with persons directly and professionally concerned with them.

5. Information obtained about participants in research should be treated as confidential.

6. The social worker should take credit only for work actually done in connection with scholarly and research endeavors and credit contributions made by others.

II. The Social Worker's Ethical Responsibility to Clients

F. Primacy of Clients' Interests - The social worker's primary responsibility is to clients.

1. The social worker should serve clients with devotion, loyalty, determination, and the maximum application of professional skill and competence.

2. The social worker should not exploit relationships with clients for personal advantage.

3. The social worker should not practice, condone, facilitate or collaborate with any form of discrimination on the

basis of race, color, sex, sexual orientation, age, religion, national origin, marital status, political belief, mental or physical handicap, or any other preference or personal characteristic, condition or status.

4. The social worker should not condone or engage in any dual or multiple relationships with clients or former clients in which there is a risk of exploitation of or potential harm to the client. The social worker is responsible for setting clear, appropriate, and culturally sensitive boundaries.

5. The social worker should under no circumstances engage in sexual activities with clients.

6. The social worker should provide clients with accurate and complete information regarding the extent and nature of the services available to them.

7. The social worker should apprise clients of their risks, rights, opportunities, and obligations associated with social service to them.

8. The social worker should seek advice and counsel of colleagues and supervisors whenever such consultation is in the best interest of clients.

9. The social worker should terminate service to clients, and professional relationships with them, when such service and relationships are no longer required or no longer serve the clients' needs or interests.

10. The social worker should withdraw services precipitously only under unusual circumstances, giving careful consideration to all factors in the situation and taking care to minimize possible adverse effects.

11. The social worker who anticipates the termination or interruption of service to clients should notify clients promptly and seek the transfer, referral, or continuation of service in relation to the clients' needs and preferences.

G. Rights and Prerogatives of Clients - The social worker should make every effort to foster maximum self-determination on the part of clients.

1. When the social worker must act on behalf of a client who has been adjudged legally incompetent, the social worker should safeguard the interests and rights of that client.

2. When another individual has been legally authorized to act in behalf of a client, the social worker should deal with that person always with the client's best interest in mind.

3. The social worker should not engage in any action that violates or diminishes the civil or legal rights of clients.

H.   Confidentiality and Privacy - The social worker should respect the privacy of clients and hold in confidence all information obtained in the course of professional service.

1. The social worker should share with others confidences revealed by clients, without their consent, only for compelling professional reasons.

2. The social worker should inform clients fully about the limits of confidentiality in a given situation, the purposes for which information is obtained, and how it may be used.

3. The social worker should afford clients reasonable access to any official social work records concerning them.

4. When providing clients with access to records, the social worker should take due care to protect the confidences of others contained in those records.

5. The social worker should obtain informed consent of clients before taping, recording, or permitting third party observation of their activities.

I.   Fees - When setting fees, the social worker should ensure that they are fair, reasonable, considerate, and commensurate with the service performed and with due regard for the clients' ability to pay.

1. The social worker should not accept anything of value for making a referral.

III.   The Social Worker's Ethical Responsibility to Colleagues

J.   Respect, Fairness, and Courtesy - The social worker should treat colleagues with respect, courtesy, fairness, and good faith.

1. The social worker should cooperate with colleagues to promote professional interests and concerns.

2. The social worker should respect confidences shared by colleagues in the course of their professional relationships and transactions.

3. The social worker should create and maintain conditions of practice that facilitate ethical and competent professional performance by colleagues.
4. The social worker should treat with respect, and represent accurately and fairly, the qualifications, views, and findings of colleagues and use appropriate channels to express judgements on these matters.
5. The social worker who replaces or is replaced by a colleague in professional practice should act with consideration for the interest, character, and reputation of that colleague.
6. The social worker should not exploit a dispute between a colleague and employers to obtain a position or otherwise advance the social worker's interest.
7. The social worker should seek arbitration or mediation when conflicts with colleagues require resolution for compelling professional reasons.
8. The social worker should extend to colleagues of other professions the same respect and cooperation that is extended to social work colleagues.
9. The social worker who serves as an employer, supervisor, or mentor to colleagues should make orderly and explicit arrangements regarding the conditions of their continuing professional relationship.
10. The social worker who has the responsibility for employing and evaluating the performance of other staff members, should fulfill such responsibility in a fair, considerate, and equitable manner, on the basis of clearly enunciated criteria.
11. The social worker who has the responsibility for evaluating the performance of employees, supervisees, or students should share evaluations with them.
12. The social worker should not use a professional position vested with power, such as that of employer, supervisor, teacher, or consultant, to his or her advantage or to exploit others.
13. The social worker who has direct knowledge of a social work colleague's impairment due to personal problems, psychosocial distress, substance abuse, or mental health difficulties should consult with that colleague and assist the colleague in taking remedial action.

    K.   Dealing with Colleagues' Clients - The social worker has the responsibility to relate to the clients of colleagues with full professional consideration.

        1. The social worker should not assume professional responsibility for the clients of another agency or a colleague without appropriate communication with that agency or colleague.

        2. The social worker who serves the clients of colleagues, during a temporary absence or emergency, should serve those clients with the same consideration as that afforded any client.

IV. The Social Worker's Ethical Responsibility to Employers and Employing Organizations

    L.   Commitments to Employing Organization - The social worker should adhere to commitments made to the employing organization.

        1. The social worker should work to improve the employing agency's policies and procedures, and the efficiency and effectiveness of its services.

        2. The social worker should not accept employment or arrange student field placements in an organization which is currently under public sanction by NASW for violating personnel standards, or imposing limitations on or penalties for professional actions on behalf of clients.

        3. The social worker should act to prevent and eliminate discrimination in the employing organization's work assignments and in its employment policies and practices.

        4. The social worker should use with scrupulous regard, and only for the purpose for which they are intended, the resources of the employing organization.

V. The Social Worker's Ethical Responsibility to the Social Work Profession

    M. Maintaining the Integrity of the Profession - The social worker should uphold and advance the values, ethics, knowledge, and mission of the profession.

        1. The social worker should protect and enhance the dignity and integrity of the profession and should be responsible and vigorous in discussion and criticism of the profession.

2. The social worker should take action through appropriate channels against unethical conduct by any other member of the profession.
3. The social worker should act to prevent the unauthorized and unqualified practice of social work.
4. The social worker should make no misrepresentation in advertising as to qualifications, competence, service, or results to be achieved.

N. Community Service - The social worker should assist the profession in making social services available to the general public.

1. The social worker should contribute time and professional expertise to activities that promote respect for the utility, the integrity, and the competence of the social work profession.
2. The social worker should support the formulation, development, enactment and implementation of social policies of concern to the profession.

O. Development of Knowledge - The social worker should take responsibility for identifying, developing, and fully utilizing knowledge for professional practice.

1. The social worker should base practice upon recognized knowledge relevant to social work.
2. The social worker should critically examine, and keep current with emerging knowledge relevant to social work.
3. The social worker should contribute to the knowledge base of social work and share research knowledge and practice wisdom with colleagues.

VI. The Social Worker's Ethical Responsibility to Society

P. Promoting the General Welfare - The social worker should promote the general welfare of society.

1. The social worker should act to prevent and eliminate discrimination against any person or group on the basis of race, color, sex, sexual orientation, age, religion, national origin, marital status, political belief, mental or physical handicap, or any other preference or personal characteristic, condition, or status.
2. The social worker should act to ensure that all persons have access to the resources, services, and opportunities which they require.

3. The social worker should act to expand choice and opportunity for all persons, with special regard for disad-
   vantaged or oppressed groups and persons.
4. The social worker should promote conditions that encourage respect for the diversity of cultures which constitute
   American society.
5. The social worker should provide appropriate professional services in public emergencies.
6. The social worker should advocate changes in policy and
   legislation to improve social conditions and to promote
   social justice.
7. The social worker should encourage informed participation by the public in shaping social policies and institutions.

Appendix E

An Illustrative
Informed Consent Statement
Used in an Outpatient Practice

PATIENT INFORMATION
Dr. _____

This provides some basic information about psychological treatment. Please read and sign at the bottom to indicate that you have reviewed this information.

LENGTH OF TREATMENT

Psychotherapy typically involves regular sessions, usually 50 minutes in length. Duration of treatment varies depending on the nature of the problem and your individual needs.

CONFIDENTIALITY

Information shared with a psychologist is kept strictly condfidential and is not disclosed without your written permission. However, confidentiality is not guaranteed in cases of (a) danger to yourself or others (e.g., homicide or suicide), or (b) situations in which children are endangered (e.g., sexual or physical abuse or neglect).

FEE POLICIES

The ordinary charge for an individual or joint therapy session is $80.00. If you need to cancel an appointment, 24 hours notice is appreciated. Otherwise, cancellation charges may be incurred; please be aware that insurance carriers will not cover cancellation charges.

If you carry mental health insurance coverage, our office will bill your carrier and assist with insurance reimbursement. However, please be aware that charges are the patient's responsibility. In addition, any copayment necessary should be made at the time of the session.

Telephone consultations, preparation of records, and correspondence are billed pro-rata if substantial time is required. Court testimony and psychological testing charges are variable; please discuss these as necessary.

Our office reserves the right to engage the services of a collection agency in the event of unpaid balances; charges for collection efforts also become the patient's responsibility.

EMERGENCIES

When Dr. _____ is unavailable, arrangements can be made for coverage or telephone contact as necessary. The after-hours telephone number at the office is _____.

PHYSICIAN CONTACT

Physical and psychological symptoms often interact, and we encourage you to seek medical consultation if warranted. In addition, medication may sometimes be helpful for psychological disorders. When appropriate, referral for psychiatric consultation can be arranged.

FREEDOM TO WITHDRAW

You have the right to end therapy at any time and are obligated only to pay for completed sessions. If you wish, Dr. _____ will provide you with names of other qualified psychotherapists.

INFORMED CONSENT

I have read and understood the preceding statements, have had the opportunity to ask questions about them, and agree to begin treatment with Dr. _____.

Name_____ Date_____

References

Abraham v. Zaslow, Docket No. 245862 (Sup. Ct. Santa Clara County, Oct. 26, 1970). Reported in Glenn R. (1974).

American Association for Marriage and Family Therapy. (1991). *Code of Ethics.* Washington, DC: Author.

American Association of State Psychology Boards. (1985). *Guidelines for Computer Based Assessment and Interpretation.* New York: Author.

American Educational Research Association, American Psychological Association, & National Council on Measurement in Education. (1985). *Standards for Educational and Psychological Testing.* Washington, DC: American Psychological Association.

American Psychiatric Association. (1993). *The Principles of Medical Ethics With Annotations Especially Applicable to Psychiatry.* Washington, DC: Author.

American Psychiatric Association. (1994). *Diagnostic and Statistical Manual of Mental Disorders* (4th ed.). Washington, DC: Author.

American Psychological Association. (1981). *Specialty Guidelines for the Delivery of Services by Clinical Psychologists.* Washington, DC: Author.

American Psychological Association. (1982). *Ethical Principles in the Conduct of Research With Human Participants.* Washington, DC: Author.

American Psychological Association. (1986). *Guidelines for Computer Based Tests and Interpretations.* Washington, DC: Author.

American Psychological Association. (1987). General guidelines for providers of psychological services. *American Psychologist, 42,* 712-723.

American Psychological Association. (1992). Ethical principles of psychologists and code of conduct. *American Psychologist, 44,* 1597-1611.

American Psychological Association. (1994). *Publication Manual of the American Psychological Association* (4th ed.). Washington, DC: Author.

Applebaum, P. S. (1983). Paternalism and the role of the mental health lawyer. *Hospital and Community Psychiatry, 34,* 211-212.

Applebaum, P. S. (1985). Tarasoff and the clinician: Problems in fulfilling the duty to protect. *American Journal of Psychiatry, 142,* 425-429.

Applebaum, P. S. (1990). The parable of the forensic psychiatrist: Ethics and the problem of doing harm. *International Journal of Law and Psychiatry, 13,* 249-259.

Applebaum, P. S. (1993). Legal liability and managed care. *American Psychologist, 48,* 251-257.

Ascher, L. M., & Turner, R. M. (1980). A comparison of two methods for the administration of paradoxical intention. *Behavior Research and Treatment, 18,* 121-126.

Beauchamp, T. L., & Childress, J. F. (1979). Principles of biomedical ethics. New York: Oxford University Press.

Beck, J. (1982). When the patient threatens violence: An empirical study of clinical practice after Tarasoff. *Bulletin of the American Academy of Psychiatry and the Law, 10,* 189-201.

Beier, E. G., & Young, D. (1984). *The Silent Language of Psychotherapy* (2nd ed.). Chicago: Aldine.

Bennett, B. E., Bryant, B. K., VandenBos, G. R., & Greenwood, A. (1990). *Professional Liability and Risk Management.* Washington, DC: American Psychological Association.

Bentham, J. (1948). *An Introduction to the Principles of Morals and Legislation.* New York: Hafar Publishing. (Original work published 1863)

Berman, A. L., & Cohen-Sandler, R. (1983). Suicide and malpractice: Expert testimony and the standard of care. *Professional Psychology: Research and Practice, 14,* 6-19.

Berndt, D. J. (1983). Ethical and professional considerations in psychological assessment. *Professional Psychology: Research and Practice, 14,* 580-587.

Bernstein, B. L., & LeComte, C. (1981). Licensure and psychology: Alternative directions. *Professional Psychology, 12,* 200-208.

Bersoff, D. (1976). Psychologists as protectors and policemen: New roles as a result of Tarasoff? *Professional Psychology, 7,* 267-273.

Bouhoutsos, J., Holroyd, J., Lerman, H., Forer, B. R., & Greenberg, M. (1983). Sexual intimacy between psychotherapists and patients. *Professional Psychology: Research and Practice, 14,* 185-196.

Brodsky, S. L. (1991). *Testifying in Court: Guidelines and Maxims for the Expert Witness.* Washington, DC: American Psychological Association.

Butz, R. A. (1985). Reporting child abuse and confidentiality in counseling: Implications for social work. *Social Casework, 66,* 83-90.

Campbell, D. T., & Stanley, J. C. (1963). *Experimental and Quasi-Experimental Designs for Research.* Chicago: Rand McNally.

Candee, D. (1985). Classical ethics and live patient simulations in the moral education of health care professionals. In M. W. Berkowitz & F. Oser (Eds.), *Moral Education: Theory and Application* (pp. 297-318). Hillsdale, NJ: Lawrence Erlbaum.

Caplan, A. (1982). On privacy and confidentiality in social science research. In T. R. Beauchamp, R. R. Faden, R. J. Wallace, & L. Walters (Eds.), *Ethical Issues in Social Science Research* (pp. 315-325). Baltimore, MD: Johns Hopkins.

Caruth, E. G. (1985). Secret bearer or secret barer. *Contemporary Psychoanalysis, 4,* 548-562.

Cohen, R. J. (1979). *Malpractice: A Guide for Mental Health Professionals.* New York: The Free Press.

Cohen, R. J., & Mariano, W. E. (1982). *Legal Guidebook in Mental Health.* New York: The Free Press.

Corey, G., Corey, M. S., & Callanan, P. (1988). *Issues and Ethics in the Helping Professions* (3rd ed.). Monterey, CA: Brooks/Cole.

Dawson, C. S. (1981). *Truthtelling, Paternalism, and Autonomy in Psychotherapy.* Unpublished doctoral dissertation, California School of Professional Psychology, Berkeley, CA.

DeKraii, M. B., & Sales, B. D. (1984). Confidential communications of psychotherapists. *Psychotherapy, 21,* 293-318.

Dimatteo, R. M., & Hendricks, S. F. (1982). *Interpersonal Issues in Health Care.* New York: Academic Press.

Division of Psychology and Law. (1991). *Guidelines for the Practice of Forensic Psychology.* Washington, DC: Author.

Drew, J., Stoeckle, J. D., & Billings, J. A. (1983). Tips, status, and sacrifice: Gift giving in the doctor-patient relationship. *Social Science and Medicine, 17,* 399-404.

Dubin, S. S. (1972). Obsolescence or life-long education: A choice for the professional. *American Psychologist, 27,* 486-496.

Erickson, S. H. (1990). Counseling irresponsible AIDS patients: Guidelines for decision making. *Journal of Counseling and Development, 68,* 454-455.

Ethics Committee of the American Psychological Association. (1988). Trends in ethics cases, common pitfalls, and published resources. *American Psychologist, 43,* 564-572.

Everstine, L., Everstine, D., Haymann, G., True, R., Frey, D. E., Johnson, H., & Seiden, R. (1980). Privacy and confidentiality in psychotherapy. *American Psychologist, 35,* 828-840.

Faden, R., & Beauchamp, T. (1986). *Informed Consent: History, Theory and Implementation.* New York: Oxford.

Faust, D. (1986). Research on human judgment and its application to clinical practice. *Professional Psychology: Research and Practice, 17,* 420-430.

Faustman, W. (1982). Legal and ethical issues in debt collection strategies of professional psychologists. *Professional Psychology: Research and Practice, 13,* 208-214.

Felthous, A. (1989). The ever-confusing jurisprudence of the psychotherapist's duty to protect. *Journal of Psychiatry & Law, 17,* 575-594.

Fretz, B., & Mills, D. (1980). *Licensing and Certification of Psychologists and Counselors.* San Francisco: Jossey-Bass.

Freudenberger, H. (1982). Burnout and stress in mental health providers. In G. VandenBos (Ed.), *Professionals in Distress* (pp. 135-152). Washington, DC: American Psychological Association.

FTC demands end to ad, fee-splitting restrictions. (1988). *APA Monitor,* p. 18.

Garb, H. N. (1991). The trained psychologist as expert witness. *Professional Psychology: Research and Practice, 37,* 451-467.

Gaylin, W. (1982). The competence of children: No longer all or none. *Hastings Center Report, 12,* 33-38.

George, J. C. (1985). Hedlund paranoia. *Journal of Clinical Psychology, 41,* 291-294.

Geraty, R. D., Hendren, R., & Flaa, C. J. (1992). Ethical perspectives on managed care as it relates to child and adolescent psychiatry. *Journal of the American Academy of Child and Adolescent Psychiatry, 31,* 398-402.

Gerts, B. (1981). *The Moral Rules.* New York: Ballantine.

Goldberg, C. (1977). *Therapeutic Partnership: Ethical Concerns in Psychotherapy.* New York: Springer.

Golding, S. L. (1990). Mental health professionals and the courts: The ethics of expertise. *International Journal of Law and Psychiatry, 13,* 281-307.

Gomes-Schwartz, B., Hadley, S. W., & Strupp, H. (1978). Individual therapy and behavior therapy. *Annual Review of Psychology, 29,* 435-471.

Goodstein, L. (1983). The correct policy on co-payments. *APA Monitor,* p. 5.

Gross, S. J. (1978). The myth of professional licensing. *American Psychologist, 33,* 1009-1016.

Groth-Marnat, G. (1984). *Handbook of Psychological Assessment.* New York: Van Nostrand Reinhold.

Haas, L. J. (1993). Competence and quality in the performance of forensic psychologists. *Ethics and Behavior, 3,* 251-266.

Haas, L. J., & Cummings, N. A. (1991). Managed outpatient mental health plans: Clinical, ethical and practical guidelines for participation. *Professional Psychology: Research and Practice, 22,* 45-51.

Haas, L. J., & Hall, J. H. (1990). Impaired or unethical? Issues for colleagues and ethics committees. *The Register Report, 3,* 2-5.

Haas, L. J., Malouf, J. L., & Mayerson, N. H. (1986). Ethical dilemmas in psychological practice: Results of a national survey. *Professional Psychology: Research and Practice, 17,* 316-321.

Hall, J. E., & Hare-Mustin, R. T. (1983). Sanctions and the diversity of ethical complaints against psychologists. *American Psychologist, 38,* 714-729.

Hare-Mustin, R. T., Maracek, J., Kaplan, A., & Liss-Levinson, N. (1979). Rights of clients, responsibilities of therapists. *American Psychologist, 34,* 3-16.

Hathaway, S. R., & McKinley, J. C. (1943). *Minnesota Multiphasic Personality Inventory.* Minneapolis, MN: The Psychological Corporation.

Hathaway, S. R., & McKinley, J. C. (1989). *Minnesota Multiphasic Personality Inventory-2.* Minneapolis, MN: University of Minnesota Press.

Hills, H. I., Gruszkos, J. R., & Strong, S. R. (1985). Attribution and the double bind in paradoxical interventions. *Psychotherapy, 22,* 779-785.

Hoffman, I. (1979). Psychological versus medical psychotherapy. *Professional Psychology, 10,* 571-595.

Holder, A. (1985). *Legal Issues in Pediatrics and Adolescent Medicine.* New Haven: Yale University Press.

Horst, E. A. (1989). Dual relationships between psychologists and clients in rural and urban areas. *Journal of Rural Community Psychology, 10,* 15-24.

Hunsley, J. (1988). Conceptions and misconceptions about the context of paradoxical therapy. *Professional Psychology: Research and Practice, 19,* 553-559.

Jablonski v. United States, 712 F.2d 391 (9th Cir. 1983).

Jagim, R. D., Wittman, W., & Noll, J. (1978). Mental health professionals' attitudes toward confidentiality, privilege, and third-party disclosure. *Professional Psychology, 9,* 458-466.

Jennings, F. L. (1992). Ethics of rural practice. *Psychotherapy in Private Practice, 10,* 85-104.

Jonsen, A. R., Siegler, M., & Winslade, W. J. (1982). *Clinical Ethics.* New York: Macmillan.

Kahneman, D., & Tversky, A. (1981). The framing of decisions and the psychology of choice. *Science, 211,* 453-458.

Kahneman, D., & Tversky, A. (1984). Choices, values, and frames. *American Psychologist, 39,* 341-350.

Kalichman, S. C., & Craig. M. E. (1991). Professional psychologists' decisions to report suspected child abuse: Clinical and situational influences. *Professional Psychology, 22,* 84-89.

Kane, M. T. (1982). The validity of licensure examinations. *American Psychologist, 37,* 911-918.

Kaplan, H. S., Sager, C. J., & Schiavo, R. C. (1985). Editorial: Aids and the sex therapist. *Journal of Sex and Marital Therapy, 11,* 210-214.

Karpel, M. (1980). Family secrets: I. Conceptual and ethical issues in the relational context. II. Ethical and practical considerations in therapeutic management. *Family Process, 19,* 295-306.

Kaufman, M. (1991). Post-Tarasoff legal developments and the mental health literature. *Bulletin of the Menninger Clinic, 55,* 308-322.

Keeton, W. P. (Ed.). (1984). *Prosser and Keeton on the Law of Torts* (5th ed.). St. Paul, MN: West.

Kegeles, S., Catania, J., & Coates, T. (1988). Intentions to communicate positive HIV-antibody status to sex partners [Letter to the editor]. *Journal of the American Medical Association, 259,* 216-217.

Keith-Spiegel, P. (1977). The violation of ethical principles due to ignorance or poor professional judgment versus willful disregard. *Professional Psychology, 8,* 288-296.

Keith-Spiegel, P., & Koocher, G. P. (1985). *Ethics in Psychology: Professional Standards and Cases.* New York: Random House.

King, J. H. (1986). *The Law of Medical Malpractice*. St. Paul, MN: West.

Kinzie, J. D., Holmes, J. L., & Arent, J. (1985). Patients' release of medical records. *Hospital and Community Psychiatry, 36,* 843-847.

Knapp, S., & VandeCreek, L. (1982). Tarasoff: Five years later. *Professional Psychology, 13,* 511-516.

Knapp, S., & VandeCreek, L. (1987). *Privileged Communications in the Mental Health Professions.* New York: Van Nostrand Reinhold.

Knapp, S., & VandeCreek, L. (1990). *What Every Therapist Should Know About AIDS.* Sarasota, FL: Professional Resource Exchange.

Laliotis, D. A., & Grayson, J. H. (1985). Psychologist heal thyself: What is available for the impaired psychologist? *American Psychologist, 40,* 84-96.

Levine, M. L., & Lyon-Levine, M. (1984). Ethical conflicts at the interface of advocacy and psychiatry. *Hospital and Community Psychiatry, 35,* 665-666.

Lowman, R. (1991). Special section on managed mental health care. *Professional Psychology: Research and Practice, 22,* 5-59.

Macklin, R. (1991). HIV infected psychiatric patients: Beyond confidentiality. *Ethics and Behavior, 1,* 3-20.

Masters, W. E. L., & Johnson, V. (1988). *Crisis: Heterosexual Behavior in the Age of AIDS.* New York: Grove.

Matarazzo, J. D. (1986). Computerized clinical psychological test interpretations: Unvalidated plus all mean and no sigma. *American Psychologist, 4,* 14-24.

McGuire, J. M., Toal, P., & Blau, B. (1985). The adult clients' perception of confidentiality in the therapeutic relationship. *Professional Psychology: Research and Practice, 16,* 375-384.

Medical Information Bureau. (1993). *Your Rights to Your File.* Boston, MA: Author.

Melton, G. B. (1981). Children's participation in treatment planning: Psychological and legal issues. *Professional Psychology: Research and Practice, 12,* 246-252.

Melton, G. B., Petrila, J., Poythress, N. G., & Slogobin, C. (1987). *Psychological Evaluations for the Courts.* New York: Guilford.

Mills, D. (1984). Ethics education and adjudication in psychology. *American Psychologist, 39,* 669-675.

Monahan, J. (Ed.). (1980). *Who Is the Client?: The Ethics of Psychological Intervention in the Criminal Justice System.* Washington, DC: American Psychological Association.

National Association of Social Workers. (1993). *Code of Ethics.* Washington, DC: Author.

Norcross, J. C., & Prochaska, J. O. (1983). Psychotherapists' perspectives on treating themselves and their clients for psychic distress. *Professional Psychology: Research and Practice, 14,* 642-655.

Patel, V. L., & Groen, G. J. (1991). The general and specific nature of medical expertise: A critical look. In K. A. Ericsson & J. Smith (Eds.), *Toward a General Theory of Expertise: Prospects and Limits* (pp. 93-125). New York: Cambridge University Press.

Peck v. The Counseling Service of Addison County, 499 A. 2d 422 (Vt. 1985).

Pellegrino, E. D. (1979). Toward a reconstruction of medical morality: The primacy of the act of profession and the fact of illness. *The Journal of Medicine and Philosophy, 4,* 32-56.

Petersen v. State, 671 P.2d 230 (Wa. 1983).

Peterson, D. R., & Bry, B. H. (1980). Dimensions of perceived competence in professional psychology. *Professional Psychology, 11,* 965-971.

Petrila, J. P., & Sadoff, R. L. (1992). Confidentiality and the family as caregiver. *Hospital and Community Psychiatry, 43,* 136-139.

P. L. 93-380. (1974). The family educational rights and privacy act (The Buckley Amendment). *United States Code.* Washington, DC: Government Printing Office.

Plotkin, R. (1981). When rights collide: Parents, children and consent to treatment. *Journal of Pediatric Psychology, 6,* 121-130.

Rest, J. R. (1982). A psychologist looks at the teaching of ethics--moral development and moral education. *The Hastings Center Report, 12,* 29-36.

Rohrbaugh, T. (1982). Varieties of paradoxical therapy. *Professional Psychology: Research and Practice, 12,* 125-132.

Roll, S., & Millen, L. (1978). On violating an ethical injunction: Accepting friends as clients. *Professional Psychology, 14,* 361-372.

Roth, L. H., Wolford, J., & Meisel, A. (1980). Patient access to records, tonic or toxin? *American Journal of Psychiatry, 137,* 592-596.

Roy, J., & Freeman, L. (1976). *Betrayal: Based on the Personal Account of Julie Ray.* New York: Stein & Day.

Rubanowitz, D. E. (1987). Public attitudes toward psychotherapist-client confidentiality. *Professional Psychology: Research and Practice, 18,* 613-618.

Ryabik, J. E., Olson, K. R., & Kleim, D. M. (1984). Ethical issues in computerized psychological assessment. *Professional Practice of Psychology, 5,* 31-39.

Schetky, D. H., & Cavanaugh, J. L. (1982). Child psychiatric practice: Psychiatric malpractice. *Journal of the American Academy of Child Psychiatry, 21,* 521-526.

Schwartz, G. (1989). Confidentiality revisited. *Social Work, 34,* 223-226.

Schwitzgebel, R. L., & Schwitzgebel, R. K. (1980). *Law and Psychological Practice.* New York: Wiley.

Sell, J. M., Gottlieb, M. C., & Schoenfield, L. (1986). Ethical considerations of social/romantic relationships with present and former clients. *Professional Psychology: Research and Practice, 17,* 504-508.

Shapiro, D. L. (1990). Problems encountered in the preparation and presentation of expert testimony. In E. Margenau (Ed.), *The Encyclopedic Handbook of Private Practice* (pp. 739-758). New York: Gardner.

Shapiro, D. L. (1992). Ethical problems in the suppression of data. *Forensic Reports, 5,* 163-168.

Sonne, J. L., & Pope, K. S. (1991). Treating victims of therapist-patient sexual involvement. *Psychotherapy, 28,* 174-187.

Stockman, A. F. (1990). Dual relationships in rural mental health practice: An ethical dilemma. *Journal of Rural Community Psychology, 11,* 31-45.

Stromberg, C. (1992, August). *Managed Care: How to Practice Ethically.* Paper presented at American Psychological Association Annual Convention, Washington, DC.

Suisson, E. L., VandeCreek, L., & Knapp, S. (1987). Thorough record keeping: A good defense in a litigious era. *Professional Psychology: Research and Practice, 18,* 498-502.

Swenson, E. (1986). Legal liability for a patient's suicide. *Journal of Psychiatry & Law, 14,* 409-434.

Szasz, T. (1986). The case against suicide prevention. *American Psychologist, 41,* 806-812.

Tarasoff v. Board of Regents of the University of California, 551 P.2d 334 (Cal. 1976).

VandeCreek, L., & Knapp, S. (1993). *Tarasoff and Beyond: Legal and Clinical Considerations in the Treatment of Life-Endangering Patients* (rev. ed.). Sarasota, FL: Professional Resource Press.

VandeCreek, L., Knapp S., & Herzog, C. (1987). Malpractice risks in the treatment of dangerous patients. *Psychotherapy, 24,* 145-153.

VandenBos, G., & Duthie, R. (1986). Confronting and supporting colleagues in distress. In R Kilburg, P. Nathan, & R. Thoreson (Eds.), *Professionals in Distress: Issues, Syndromes, and Solutions in Psychology* (pp. 211-232). Washington, DC: American Psychological Association.

Webster, N. (1956). *Webster's New Twentieth Century Dictionary, 2nd Edition.* New York: World Publishing Co.

Weissman, M. L. (1991). Child custody evaluations: Fair and unfair professional practices. *Behavioral Sciences and the Law, 9,* 469-476.

Weithorn, L. A. (1983). Involving children in decisions affecting their own welfare. In G. Melton, G. Koocher, & M. Saks (Eds.), *Children's Competence to Consent* (pp. 235-260). New York: Plenum.

Wickline v. State of California, 228 Cal. 661 (Cal. Ct. App. 1986).

Wiens, A. (1983). Toward a conceptualization of competency assurance. *Professional Practice of Psychology, 4*(2), 1-15.

Wright, R. (1981). Psychologists and professional liability (malpractice) insurance: A retrospective review. *American Psychologist, 36,* 1485-1493.

Index

N

Negligence, 53, 91 (**see also** Impaired professionals)
Nonmaleficence vs. convenience, 95

P

Paradoxical interventions, 14
Paternalism, 85-96
    definition of, 86
    nonmaleficence and, 95
    protection of others and, 90-94
    withholding information and, 94-95
Practicality, 17
Preferred provider organizations (PPOs), 107
The Principles of Medical Ethics With Annotations
        Especially Applicable to Psychiatry, American
        Psychiatric Association, 21, 35, 59, 114, 118,
        123, 136, 138, 152-153, 179, 205-214
Privacy, 33-34 (**see also** Confidentiality; Privilege)
Privilege, 33, 35-36
Professional renewal, 183-189
Protection of others and paternalism, 90-94 (**see also**
        Tarasoff decision)
Prudence, 18
Psychscan, 186
Public statements, 149-157
    about general topics, 153-154
    guidelines, 156-157
    about oneself, 150-153
    about specific topics, 154-155

R

Radio talk shows (**see** Public statements)
Record keeping, 125-136
    audience for, 126-129

T

U

V

If You Found This Book Useful . . .

You might want to know more about our other titles.

If you would like to receive our latest catalog, please return this form:

Name:_____
(Please Print)

Address:_____

Address:_____

City/State/Zip:_____

Telephone:(_____)_____

I am a:

_____ Psychologist   _____ Mental Health Counselor
_____ Psychiatrist   _____ Marriage and Family Therapist
_____ School Psychologist   _____ Psychiatric Nurse
_____ Clinical Social Worker   _____ Not in Mental Health Field
                                            _____ Other:_____

◆   ◆   ◆

Professional Resource Press
P.O. Box 15560
Sarasota, FL 34277-1560

Telephone # 941-366-7913
FAX # 941-366-7971

Add A Colleague To Our Mailing List . . .

If you would like us to send our latest catalog to one of your colleagues, please return this form.

Name:_____
(Please Print)

Address:_____

Address:_____

City/State/Zip:_____

Telephone:(_____)_____

I am a:

_____ Psychologist   _____ Mental Health Counselor
_____ Psychiatrist   _____ Marriage and Family Therapist
_____ School Psychologist   _____ Psychiatric Nurse
_____ Clinical Social Worker   _____ Not in Mental Health Field
                                              _____ Other:_____

◆   ◆   ◆

Professional Resource Press
P.O. Box 15560
Sarasota, FL 34277-1560

Telephone # 941-366-7913
FAX # 941-366-7971

Add A Colleague To Our Mailing List . . .

If you would like us to send our latest catalog to one of your colleagues, please return this form.

Name:_____
        (Please Print)

Address:_____

Address:_____

City/State/Zip:_____

Telephone:(_____)_____

I am a:

_____ Psychologist	_____ Mental Health Counselor
_____ Psychiatrist	_____ Marriage and Family Therapist
_____ School Psychologist	_____ Psychiatric Nurse
_____ Clinical Social Worker	_____ Not in Mental Health Field
	_____ Other:_____

◆   ◆   ◆

Professional Resource Press
P.O. Box 15560
Sarasota, FL 34277-1560

Telephone # 941-366-7913
FAX # 941-366-7971

Add A Colleague To Our Mailing List . . .

If you would like us to send our latest catalog to one of your colleagues, please return this form.

Name:_____
(Please Print)

Address:_____

Address:_____

City/State/Zip:_____

Telephone:(_____)_____

I am a:

_____ Psychologist	_____ Mental Health Counselor
_____ Psychiatrist	_____ Marriage and Family Therapist
_____ School Psychologist	_____ Psychiatric Nurse
_____ Clinical Social Worker	_____ Not in Mental Health Field
	_____ Other:_____

◆   ◆   ◆

Professional Resource Press
P.O. Box 15560
Sarasota, FL 34277-1560

Telephone # 941-366-7913
FAX # 941-366-7971